Animal Biology and Care

Second Edition

S. E. Dallas
VN, CertEd

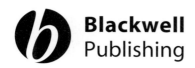
Blackwell
Publishing

Blackwell Publishing editorial offices:
Blackwell Publishing Ltd, 9600 Garsington Road,
Oxford OX4 2DQ, UK
    Tel: +44 (0)1865 776868
Blackwell Publishing Professional, 2121 State
Avenue, Ames, Iowa 50014-8300, USA
    Tel: +1 515 292 0140
Blackwell Publishing Asia Pty Ltd, 550 Swanston
Street, Carlton, Victoria 3053, Australia
    Tel: +61 (0)3 8359 1011

First edition published 2000 by Blackwell Science Ltd
Second edition published 2006 by Blackwell
Publishing Ltd

3   2008

ISBN: 978-1-4051-3795-9

Library of Congress Cataloging-in-Publication
Data
Dallas, S. E. (Sue E.)
    [Animal biology and care. Selections]
    Animal biology and care / S. E. Dallas. – 2nd
ed.
    p. cm.
    Includes bibliographical references and
index.
    ISBN-13: 978-1-4051-3795-9 (pbk. : alk.
paper)
    ISBN-10: 1-4051-3795-9 (pbk. : alk. paper)
    1. Veterinary medicine.   I. Title.
SF745. D246 2006
636.089 – dc22
2005028054

A catalogue record for this title is available from
the British Library

Set in 10 on 13 pt Times
by SNP Best-set Typesetter Ltd, Hong Kong
Printed and bound in Great Britain
by TJ International Ltd, Padstow, Cornwall

The publisher's policy is to use permanent paper
from mills that operate a sustainable forestry
policy, and which has been manufactured from
pulp processed using acid-free and elementary
chlorine-free practices. Furthermore, the publisher
ensures that the text paper and cover board used
have met acceptable environmental accreditation
standards.

For further information on Blackwell Publishing,
visit our website:
www.BlackwellVet.com

Contents

Preface

The increasing need for competence and understanding of animal care, both in the home and the work place, were the motivation for writing this book. It is intended as a foundation text for those on animal care, nurse auxiliary and veterinary care assistant courses. I hope that it will also prove of value to a wider range of readers, giving them a useful and enjoyable introduction to the background required, and the skills to develop, when considering the care of any animal.

The book seeks to provide information in a readily accessible layout, and is illustrated with line drawings and photographs. With a better understanding and knowledge of the care required by animals, injury and ill health can be better avoided or managed. The basic principles of nursing and care remain unchanged whether carried out at home, in the work place or within a veterinary practice. Methods for the control or elimination of disease are the same whether one is dealing with a single animal or a large group, for example in a kennel, cattery or animal collection.

The first edition concentrated on the biology, husbandry and care of mammals. This has now been expanded to include more detail on small mammals, birds and fish. Sections on legislation, pet travel, nutrition and parasites have also been updated and/or expanded, providing more detailed information.

The book is divided into three sections, each concentrating on a specific area:

- Section 1 – Animal biology. This introduces the reader to basic cell and tissue structure through to organ structures, systems and function.
- Section 2 – Animal health and husbandry. This takes the reader through the basic requirements for animal health, detailing welfare, care, husbandry, disease recognition and its control.
- Section 3 – Nursing. This covers the nursing procedures for an animal, both before and after professional attention from a veterinary surgeon, with an introduction to medical terminology in common use.

Many thanks go to the staff at Blackwell Publishing for their continued guidance, to family and friends, particularly Peter Roe and David Williams, for their support and encouragement throughout the writing process.

Sue Dallas
VN, CertEd

Section 1
Animal Biology

Chapter 1
Cells and Basic Tissue

Biology – the study of life and living organisms

But what is life?

This is best answered by stating what distinguishes a living organism from a non-living organism. In order to be considered alive, the following are essential:

- *Growth* – from within by a process which involves the intake of new materials from the outside and their incorporation in the internal structure of the organism.
- *Movement* – the organism is capable of moving itself or a part of itself.
- *Excretion* – the removal of the waste products of metabolism.
- *Eating* – taking in materials to maintain life and growth.
- *Responsiveness* – to stimuli in its surroundings.
- *Release of energy* – in a controlled and usable form.

> Therefore considering units of life:
>
> *Cells* form . . .
> *Tissues*, and tissues form . . .
> *Organs*, and organs have a . . .
> *Function* to perform in the living organism!

The cell is the functional unit of all tissues and has the ability to perform individually all the essential life functions. Within the various tissues of the body, the constituent cells show a wide range of specialisations. However, all cells conform to a basic model of cell structure.

The diversity of cells

All cells are not identical (Fig. 1.1) but all have the same basic features:

- Chromosomes
- Mitochondria

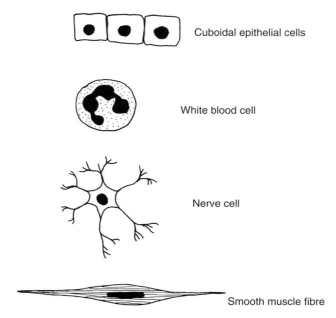

Cuboidal epithelial cells

White blood cell

Nerve cell

Smooth muscle fibre

Fig. 1.1 Diversity of cells from their basic form.

- Endoplasmic reticulum
- Ribosomes

The above are common to virtually all cells but the shape, form and contents of individual cells show much variation. The structural characteristics of a particular cell are closely related to its functions.

- *Epithelial cells* – have a shape and form that makes them most suitable for lining the surface of the body and the organs and cavities within it.
- *Glandular cells* – are responsible for producing some kind of secretion, for example mucus to lubricate between tissues.
- *Osteoblasts* – produce bone tissue.
- *Erythrocytes* (*red blood cells*) – have a shape designed to hold the red pigment haemoglobin which conveys oxygen around the body. In order to do this, they are one of the few cells in the body which no longer contain a nucleus.
- *Nerve cells* – or neurones, have slender arm-like processes which will transmit electrical impulses through the nervous system to reach the whole body.
- *Muscle cells* – are also capable of electrical activity accompanied by a muscle contraction for body movement.

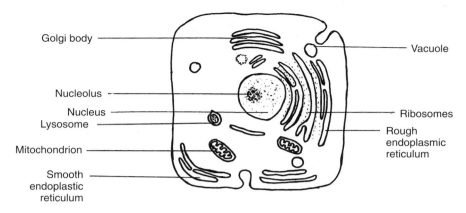

Golgi body

Vacuole

Nucleolus

Nucleus

Lysosome

Ribosomes

Rough endoplasmic reticulum

Mitochondrion

Smooth endoplastic reticulum

Fig. 1.2   Basic cell structure.

Cells

Cells have the same basic structure no matter what their function is or what organism they are found in (Fig. 1.2). Therefore the single cell which forms the body of an amoeba and the brain cell of a dog have certain features in common. All cells contain:

- A *nucleus* – to control the cell's activities
- *Cytoplasm* – a jelly-like material to support organs
- *Cell membrane* – this encloses the cytoplasm in which lies the nucleus

These three parts make up *protoplasm* – living matter.
For life, cells require:

- Food for energy
- Water (body fluid) to hydrate the cells
- Oxygen to all cells
- Suitable temperature in which to live

The nucleus

At least one nucleus is found in the cells of all organisms. The nucleus of a cell contains rod-shaped objects called *chromosomes*. These are only visible when a cell is about to divide into two. Chromosomes contain a complex chemical called *deoxyribonucleic acid (DNA)*. DNA controls the development of the features that an organism inherits from its parents. In other words, it contains the chemical 'instructions' for making an organism.

The cell membrane

The cell membrane is 0.00001 mm thick and forms the outer boundary of the cell. It is here that all exchanges take place between a cell and its surrounding environment. In a manner which is not yet fully understood, this membrane allows certain chemicals to pass in and out of the cell but prevents the passage of others (referred to as *osmosis*). As a result, the cell membranes are said to be *selectively permeable*.

The cytoplasm

The term *cytoplasm* refers to all the living substances of a cell except the nucleus. Cytoplasm is a jelly-like material containing a large number of important substances, many of which are concerned with metabolism.

- *Organelles* – are the structures visible within the cell other than the nucleus.
- *Mitochondria* – are one of the most important organelles, where chemical reactions of respiration take place. This is the release of energy for cellular function.
- *Rough endoplasmic reticulum* – has ribosomes on it that have been produced in the nucleus. Protein is synthesised here and the cell may transport it for use in the manufacture of digestive enzymes and hormones.
- *Smooth endoplasmic reticulum* – does not have ribosomes but is concerned with the synthesis and transport of lipids (fats) and steroids of body origin.
- *Ribosomes* – are granules rich in ribonucleic acid, in which protein is synthesised.
- *Centrosome* – lies near the nucleus and is made up of two *centrioles*. It is important during cell division and the formation of the cilia and flagella of certain cells (the slender projecting hairs for movement of single-celled organisms).
- *Lysosomes* – are dark round bodies containing enzymes responsible for splitting complex chemical compounds into simpler ones (known as *lysis*, meaning 'to break up') followed by digestion. They also destroy worn-out organelles within the cell. These destructive enzymes are stored in tubes in the cell called the *Golgi complex or body*.

Basic tissue

Tissues are a collection of cells and their products, which have a common fundamental function and in which one particular type of cell predominates.

- *Epithelial* – which forms a protective layer both inside and on the surface of the body. Examples of this tissue are skin, glands and the linings of the various body systems.
- *Connective* – which supports tissues and acts as a transport system to move materials vital to tissue cells around the body. Examples of this tissue are:
  (a)   loose connective tissue which surrounds organs
  (b)   dense connective tissue which has great strength and is found as tendons and ligaments
  (c)   blood which transports essential nutrients, gases, waste products, hormones and enzymes to and from all body cells
  (d)   cartilage and bone which provide shape and protection for organs and allow movement.
- *Muscular* – tissues concerned with movement of the skeleton, organ systems and the heart.
- *Nervous* – which transports messages to tissues, connecting the body as a whole for the required response.

Epithelial tissue

This tissue covers all surfaces of the body, both inside and out, be it a surface, a cavity or a tube. It is made up of a diverse group of tissues which are involved in a wide range of activities such as secretion of a special fluid, protection and absorption.

Depending on their function, the cells of this tissue will have a varied shape, structure and thickness. They are classified according to appearance:

- *Number of layers* – a single layer of these cells is called *simple epithelium*; more than one layer is called *stratified epithelium*.
- *Shape* of the cells involved.
- *Specialisations*, such as tiny hairs called cilia or special thickened surface tissue called keratin, which covers the nose and pads of the feet.
- *Glandular* – meaning it is involved in secretion. Secretions which go directly into the bloodstream are called *hormones* and are produced by glands of the *endocrine* or *ductless system*. If the gland has a duct it will secrete onto a surface and belongs to the *exocrine system*; for example, enzymes secreted by the pancreas.

The many and varied functions of epithelial tissue mean that it will take different forms. There are six main types.

Pavement – found lining surfaces involved in the transport of gases (lungs) or fluids (walls of blood vessels) (Fig. 1.3a).
Cuboidal – which lines small ducts and tubes like those of the kidney, pancreas and salivary glands of the mouth (Fig. 1.3b).
Columnar – located on highly absorbing surfaces like the small intestine for the uptake of nutrients (Fig. 1.3c).

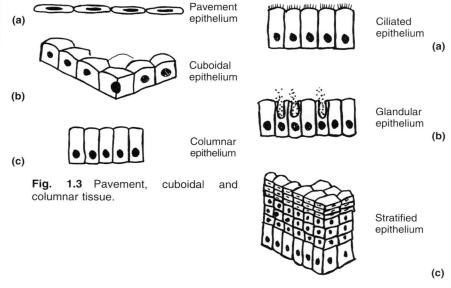

Fig. 1.3 Pavement, cuboidal and columnar tissue.

Fig. 1.4 Ciliated, glandular and stratified tissues.

Ciliated – has tiny hair-like projections in parallel rows on the surface of the cell, which beat in a wave-like manner, moving films of mucus or fluid in a particular direction. For example, in the respiratory airway (trachea), they remove unwanted inhaled materials (Fig. 1.4a).
Glandular – which secrete a special fluid containing hormones or enzymes (Fig. 1.4b).
Stratified – this type of epithelium has two or more layers of cells. Its function is mostly protection. Found lining the mouth cavity or as skin (Fig. 1.4c).

Connective tissue

This tissue binds all the other body tissues together. It supports them and acts as a transport system for the exchange of nutrients, metabolites and waste products between tissues and the circulatory system (Fig. 1.5).

Connective tissues occur in many different forms with a wide range of physical properties.

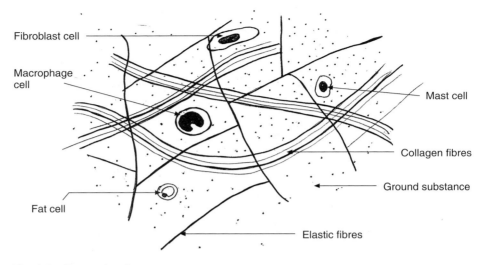

Fibroblast cell

Macrophage cell

Mast cell

Collagen fibres

Ground substance

Fat cell

Elastic fibres

Fig. 1.5 Connective tissue.

- *Loose* connective tissue acts as a type of packing material between other tissues with specific functions.
- *Dense* connective tissue provides tough support in the skin.
- *Rigid* forms of connective tissue, like cartilage and bone, support the skeleton.

Connective tissue also has functions including the storage of fat in adipose tissue, fighting infection with micro-organisms and tissue repair.

Connective tissue has two components.

(1) *Cells*:
- fibroblasts for repair and maintenance of the tissue
- fat-storing cells
- defence and immune function cells called *macrophages*.
(2) Material called *ground substance* which holds together other materials to make up tissue and looks like a semifluid gel.

Connective tissue is composed of two types of fibre.

- *Collagen* – produced by the fibroblasts, is not elastic but has great tensile strength. Tendons by which muscles are attached to bones are composed of collagen fibres.
- *Elastin* – has great elasticity and is found in ligaments which bind bones of the skeleton together.

Connective tissue can be described as a mixture of fibres in different proportions. Its efficiency in binding structures together is achieved by the special grouping of proteins in the ground substance. The particular type and abundance of fibre present depend on the stresses and strains to which the tissue is normally subjected.

Blood

This is a highly specialised tissue consisting of several types of cell suspended in a fluid medium called *plasma*. The cellular constituents consist of:

- Red blood cells (erythrocytes)
- White blood cells (leucocytes)
- Platelets (thrombocytes)

Blood has a varied structure and performs a wide range of functions. One of its main functions is that of transportation, of the red blood cells around the body and all the materials in the plasma. Blood is considered a tissue because it connects all the cells in the body together.

Live animals constantly absorb useful substances like oxygen and food, which must then be distributed throughout their bodies. They produce a continuous stream of waste materials, such as carbon dioxide, which must be removed from their bodies before they reach harmful levels. The distribution of food, oxygen and other substances throughout the body and the removal of any wastes is performed by this transport system tissue.

Composition of the blood

Fluid called *plasma* makes up about 60%. Cells and other material in transit make up the remaining 40%.

If a sample of blood (mixed with an anticoagulant to stop it clotting) was put into a centrifuge and spun to separate out the component parts, it would show at the top of the tube the fluid part (plasma), then the platelets (cell fragments), then the white blood cells and finally the red cells (Fig. 1.6).

Plasma

This is mainly water containing a variety of dissolved substances which are transported from one part of the body to another. To give a few examples, food materials (glucose, lipids and amino acids) are conveyed from the small intestine to the liver; urea from the liver to the kidneys; hormones from various ductless glands to their target organs. Cells are constantly shedding materials into the blood which flows past them and removing materials from it. Plasma provides the medium through which this continual exchange takes place.

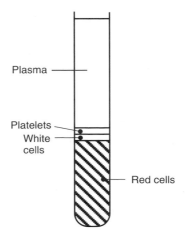

Fig. 1.6   Blood separated into layers.

PLASMA

FIBRINOGEN (protein for clotting) **plus** water, protein, glucose, lipids, amino acids, salts, enzymes, hormones and waste products

SERUM

Contains water, protein, glucose, lipids, amino acids, salts, enzymes, hormones and waste products **but** no proteins for clotting (these have been used up)

Plasma carries many more products than the diagram shows, including the plasma proteins called albumin, globulin and fibrinogen. Fibrinogen plays an important role in the process of blood clotting. When it has been used up by clot formation then the fluid part of blood seen at the site of injury is called *serum*. Therefore, serum is plasma with the fibrinogen removed. About 92% of blood is made of water and this same water can be forced into the tissues. It is then called *tissue fluid* because of its location.

It is important to realise that plasma and the tissue fluid derived from it form the environment which keeps body cells alive. In a sense, these fluids are equivalent to a pond or fish tank in which both single-celled organisms and multicelled organisms live and are supplied with their food and oxygen and into which they excrete waste.

Red blood cells (erythrocytes)

These are produced in the red or active bone marrow. The main function of red blood cells is to carry oxygen from the respiratory organ to the tissues and their structure is modified accordingly. These cells have had their nucleus removed, with the result that the cell is sunk in on each side, giving it the shape of a biconcave disc. It is surrounded by a thin elastic membrane and the interior of the cell

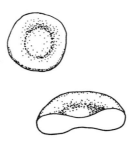

Fig. 1.7 Cross-section of a red blood cell showing its biconcave shape.

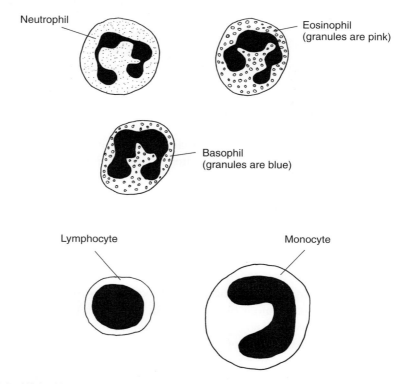

Fig. 1.8 White blood cells.

is filled with the red pigment haemoglobin which combines with and carries oxygen (Fig. 1.7).

White blood cells (leucocytes)

The white cells are fewer in number and have a very different role to play. They fall into two groups (Fig. 1.8).

Granulocytes (granules in the cytoplasm). These are produced in the bone marrow.

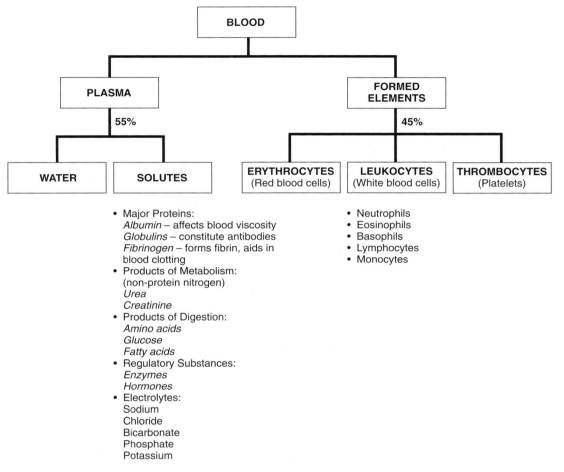

Fig. 1.9 Blood components.

- *Neutrophils* – phagocytic cells
- *Eosinophils* – respond to allergies
- *Basophils* – promote inflammation for healing of tissue

Agranulocytes (no granules in their cytoplasm). Produced in the bone marrow or lymph system.

- *Lymphocytes* – support the immune system
- *Monocytes* – phagocyte cells

Phagocyte or *phagocytic* means 'cell eater'. These cells eat or engulf other cells / materials that may be harmful and destroy them. Red cells will remain in the bloodstream to perform their role of oxygen carrier but white cells will only use the bloodstream as a transporter from their site of origin to the capillaries where they will push through the wall of the blood vessel and into the tissue spaces. Those that are phagocytic will gather in and around wounds and destroy bacteria and any other harmful material. In this manner the cells assist in 'fighting infection'.

Bone and cartilage

There are two kinds of skeletal tissue, bone and cartilage.

Bone

This tissue is closely related to connective tissue, in that it consists of cells embedded in an organic matrix (ground substance). However, this matrix is comparatively hard. The cells of bone are called *osteoblasts* and *osteoclasts*.

Cartilage

This is a dense, clear, blue/white material which provides support for the body and can be elastic or rigid. Found mainly in joints, it has no blood vessels but is covered by a membrane called the *perichondrium* from which it receives its blood supply. The cells of cartilage are called *chondroblasts*.

There are three types of cartilage:

- *Hyaline* – the cells for hyaline production are called *chondrocytes*. They lie within a hyaline matrix with collagen fibres running through. Hyaline is a smooth tissue and forms articular joint surfaces for bones and the C-shaped rings of cartilage that keep the trachea open for air passage into the lungs.
- *Fibrocartilage* – this is stronger than hyaline but with a similar base structure that contains more collagen fibres. It surrounds the articular surface of some bones, for example in the hip joint (acetabulum) and the shoulder joint (glenoid cavity), and is also found in the stifle or knee joint as pads of cartilage called *menisci*.
- *Elastic* – this has a hyaline matrix and many elastic fibres which provide its elastic properties. It is found in the ear flap (pinna) and in the larynx area of the throat.

Muscular tissue

The ability to contract is very well developed in this type of tissue. Muscle cells are usually long, thin and thread-like and are often called *fibres*. There are three main types of fibres:

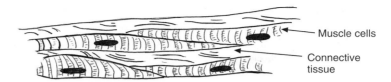

Fig. 1.10   Skeletal (striated) muscle fibre.

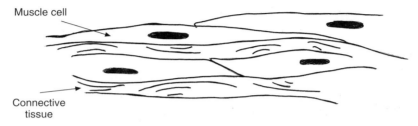

Fig. 1.11   Smooth (non-striated) muscle fibre.

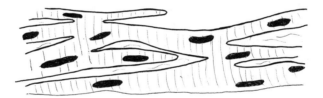

Fig. 1.12   Cardiac muscle fibre.

- *Skeletal* (also called voluntary and striated) (Fig. 1.10)
- *Smooth* (also called involuntary, non-striated and visceral) (Fig. 1.11)
- *Cardiac* (Fig. 1.12)

Skeletal muscle

Found in muscles attached to the skeleton. The cells are cylindrical and vary from about 1 mm to 5 cm in length. Since skeletal muscles respond to the will of the animal, the cells are also called *voluntary* muscle cells.

Skeletal muscles are formed of parallel muscle cells (*fibres*) held together in small bundles by connective tissue. These are collected into larger groups which are also enclosed in connective tissue and ultimately form the muscle which is surrounded by yet more connective tissue commonly called the *muscle sheath*.

When muscles are close to one another, the sheaths may thicken to form an *intermuscular septa*.

All the connective tissue within and around the muscles continues into the connective tissue of the structure to which the muscle is attached, i.e. bone.

Sometimes the muscle appears to attach directly but usually the connective tissue leaves the muscle as a fibrous band known as a *tendon* (i.e. Achilles tendon on the point of the hock) or as a fibrous sheet called an *aponeurosis* (i.e. the sheet of muscle and connective tissue called the diaphragm).

Some muscles are named according to their shape, some according to their functions and others according to their position in the body.

Under the microscope, skeletal muscle cells look striped (they have *striations*).

Smooth muscle

In direct contrast to skeletal muscle, which is specialised for relatively forceful contractions of short duration and under voluntary control, smooth muscle is specialised for continuous contractions of little force but over a greater section of muscle tissue. For example, the smooth muscle of the intestinal wall contracts in continuous rhythm, moving food through the tract by *peristaltic action*.

These fibres are spindle shaped and about 0.5 mm in length or shorter. Under the microscope they look smooth. Only small amounts of connective tissue bind them together to form sheets or layers of muscle tissue. They may also be called *involuntary* muscles because they are not controlled by the will of the animal. These fibres are found in the muscle of organs, hence the alternative name of *visceral* muscle.

Cardiac muscle

This muscle produces strong contractions using a lot of energy and is only found in the heart. The contractions are continuous. In order for this to take place, the fibres have junctions or connections with surrounding fibres which allow very rapid contractions of all nearby tissue. The cells are elongated and are the only muscle cells which frequently branch. They are held together by only very small amounts of connective tissue.

Nervous tissue

The function of this tissue is to transmit electrical messages from one part of the body to another. As a result of this, the nerve cells are interconnected in a very complex way. The cells can transmit and sometimes store information because of this complex link-up with each other.

The cells are called *neurones* (Fig. 1.13) and they connect and communicate to form pathways so that the body can respond to information received. Neurones vary in size and shape depending on where they are in the nervous system. However, all neurones have the same basic structure. They consist of a large cell body containing the nucleus surrounded by cytoplasm, with two types of processes extending from the cell body: a single axon and one or more dendrites.

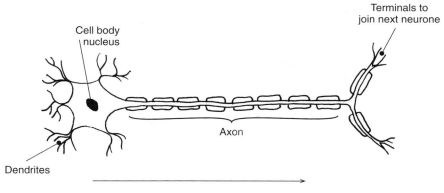

Fig. 1.13   A neurone.

Dendrites are branched, tapering processes which either end in specialised *sense receptors* (information) or form junctions (*synapses*) with neighbouring neurones from which they receive electrical stimuli, which is passed to the cells beyond.

Axons extend from the cell body as a tube-like structure of variable length, carrying stimuli or messages away to the next nerve cell.

Chapter 2
Movement of Materials Within the Body

Time now to look at the processes by which materials get into and out of cells. Exchanges can be examined under the following headings:

(1) Diffusion
(2) Osmosis
(3) Phagocytosis
(4) Active transport

Diffusion

This is the process of movement of molecules from a region where they are at a comparatively high concentration to a region where they are at a lower concentration, requiring no energy in its achievement. Diffusion will always continue until eventually the molecules are uniformly distributed throughout the system. This is very important in the movement of molecules and salts (electrolytes or ions) in and out of cells.

An example of this process is the cell's requirement for oxygen. It is continually being used up in respiration so the concentration of oxygen inside the cell will be lower than it is in the blood and tissue fluids as a result. Oxygen molecules will diffuse into the cell from outside. With carbon dioxide, the reverse is true: its concentration is highest inside the cells, where it is continually being formed. This results in carbon dioxide molecules diffusing out of the cells.

Anything that increases the concentration of a substance in the body will favour diffusion. Blood is involved here to carry away the diffused substance, so encouraging further diffusion.

Osmosis

This refers to the movement of water through a semipermeable membrane while expending no energy (Fig. 2.1).

Although the cell wall membrane is fully permeable to respiratory gases, it is not permeable to all substances. The nature of the membrane means that only molecules that are small enough will diffuse through it unimpeded. Larger molecules either penetrate slowly or not at all. The membrane is therefore called *semipermeable*, permitting the passage of some substances but not others.

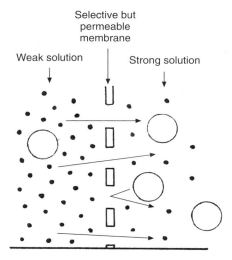

Selective but
permeable
membrane

Weak solution   Strong solution

Large molecules cannot pass through the membrane, but water passes through easily

Fig. 2.1 Osmosis.

Osmosis is really a special case of diffusion: it involves the passage of water molecules from a region of high concentration to a region of lower concentration. The concentration will be supplied by other products like salts.

Terms

Osmosis – is the diffusion of fluid through a selectively permeable membrane, from where water is in a high concentration (a *weak solution*) to where water is in a low concentration (a *strong solution*). Osmotic pressure helps to keep fluid in its correct compartment within the body.

Isotonic – refers to solutions which cause no transfer of fluid either into or out of a cell. These are the solutions most frequently used in fluid replacement in sick animals, such as 0.9% sodium chloride.

Hypertonic – these are solutions with an osmotic pressure higher than that of body fluids. If the cell is surrounded by a solution with an osmotic pressure higher than that of the cell, water passes out of the cell, causing it to shrink.

Hypotonic – these are solutions with an osmotic pressure lower than body fluid. In this case the cell is surrounded by almost pure water which allows water to enter cells by osmosis, causing the cell to swell and even to burst.

Phagocytosis

The previous headings have outlined how individual molecules cross the cell membrane; this heading covers the larger particles which also need to enter cells. This is achieved by specialised cells which are able to 'cell eat' or *phagocytose*. This process was mentioned when discussing white blood cells which take up and destroy bacteria and other particles which could be harmful to the body.

To phagocytose, the cell membrane changes shape to form a flask-like depression enclosing the particles. The neck of the depression then closes and seals itself off as a food vacuole and migrates towards the centre of the cell. The material is digested by enzymes within the cell. Any useful food products resulting from this process are absorbed into the cell cytoplasm. Phagocytosis is a selective process with the cell distinguishing between food particles and harmful materials.

Active transport

Diffusion is a purely physical process in which molecules or salts move from a region of higher to a region of lower concentration. But there are certain biological situations where the reverse happens: molecules or salts move from a region of low concentration to a region of higher concentration. They move against the *concentration gradient*. This *active transport* will only take place in a living system that is actively producing energy by respiration. It is not merely a passive barrier but a very active interface between the cell's contents and its immediate surroundings, requiring energy expenditure.

Body fluid

Dissolved in the body fluids are the essential salts called *electrolytes* or *ions*. They are called electrolytes because they carry one or more electrical charges. Those that are positively charged are called *cations*, i.e. sodium and potassium. Those that are negatively charged are called *anions*, i.e. chloride and bicarbonate.

Their role is to:

- Help control the osmotic pressure
- Assist the pH and buffer mechanisms
- Support the enzyme systems

About 60% of the body consists of fluids. It is divided into two areas:

- Intracellular – 40%
- Extracellular – 20%

Extracellular fluid is further divided into:

- *Tissue fluid* (interstitial) which bathes the tissues and cells
- *Plasma*, which is the water part of blood, needed to transport the cells, nutrients, gases, hormones and waste products

Acids and bases in the body

The acidity of a solution is expressed as its **pH** (per hydrogen). A pH of 7.0 represents neutral. A solution with a pH of less than 7.0 is acidic and the lower the figure, the higher the acidity (the greater the hydrogen ion concentration). A solution whose pH is greater than 7.0 is basic or alkaline and the higher the figure, the more basic is the solution.

The body functions within a normal range of 7.35–7.45 pH. This normal range must be maintained by the body systems at all times for the correct internal environment.

Tissue fluid and the lymphatic system

Each tissue and organ in the body contains a dense network of capillaries (blood vessels that are one cell thick). These are called the *capillary beds*. Tissue fluid is forced under pressure through the capillary walls. This process tends to occur at the artery end of the capillary bed, since blood pressure is greatest at this point.

When tissue fluid is being forced out of the capillaries, the capillary wall acts as a filter holding back red blood cells, most of the white cells and large protein molecules.

Substances which do pass through the capillary wall include:

* Water
* Oxygen
* Glucose
* Fatty acids
* Amino acids
* Vitamins and minerals
* Hormones and enzymes

Tissue fluid flows away from the capillaries and passes among the body cells, which extract oxygen, nutrients and other requirements from it and at the same time release carbon dioxide and other waste materials into it.

Lymphatic system

This is a system of open-ended tubes within the capillary bed areas, as numerous as the blood capillaries.

Lymph is tissue fluid which is not absorbed back into the bloodstream after carrying required substances to the cells. This tissue fluid drains into the open-ended tubes of the lymph system known as *lymph vessels*. The structure of these vessels is similar to that of veins, in that they have a valve system to make sure fluid only flows in one direction . The movement of lymph in these vessels is achieved by the movement of surrounding tissues which squeeze or 'milk' the fluid in the lymph vessels.

At intervals, there are *lymph nodes* (Fig. 2.2), some of which are near the surface (Fig. 2.3). These structures contain a system of narrow channels through

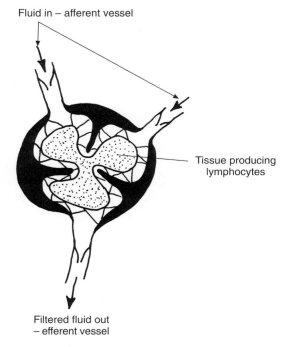

Fluid in – afferent vessel

Tissue producing lymphocytes

Filtered fluid out – efferent vessel

Fig. 2.2   Lymph node.

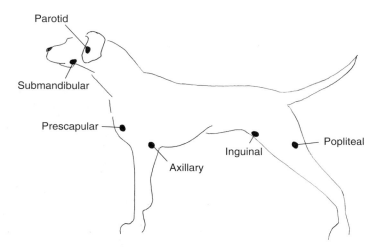

Parotid

Submandibular

Prescapular

Axillary

Inguinal

Popliteal

Fig. 2.3   Surface nodes.

which the lymph fluid will drain and be filtered. This filtering is assisted by phago-cytic white blood cells. Thus harmful substances are filtered out of the lymph, which is made safe enough to return to the circulation.

Lymph ducts are where the lymph empties into the bloodstream. From the right side of the head, neck and right forelimb, lymph drains via the right lymphatic duct. From the rest of the body, lymph drains via a collecting area called the cisterna chyli into the thoracic duct in the thorax or chest. This fluid will contain:

- Fats from the digestive system
- Water
- Electrolytes
- White blood cells
- Antibodies

Functions of the lymphatic system

- Return excess tissue fluid to the blood.
- Add lymphocytes (white blood cells) to the blood for the immune protection of the body.
- Absorb fats in the lacteals of the villi in the small intestine and carry them to the bloodstream.
- Filter out bacteria and other harmful substances via the nodes.

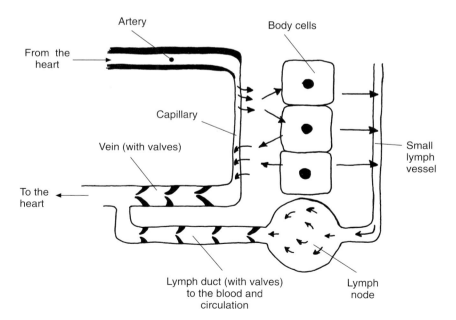

Fig. 2.4   Fluid movement from blood to lymph and back to blood.

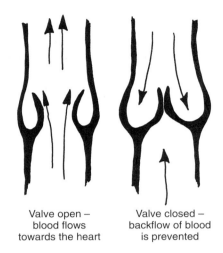

Valve open –
blood flows
towards the heart

Valve closed –
backflow of blood
is prevented

Fig. 3.1   Valve system in the veins to prevent backflow of the blood.

- Have thick muscular walls to assist with the movement of blood.
- Under high pressure, from heart muscle contractions.

Veins

- Carry blood towards the heart.
- Carry deoxygenated blood (except the pulmonary vein from the lungs to the heart).
- Have thin walls.
- Blood moved under low pressure and by action of surrounding tissues.
- Have a valve system, to prevent backflow of the blood (Fig. 3.1).

Capillaries

- Carry blood from artery to vein.
- Blood movement is very slow, to allow maximum diffusion of substances.
- Only one cell thick.
- Connects all cells and tissues, called capillary beds.
- Narrow; may only be wide enough for one blood cell at a time to pass through.

Location names for blood vessels

The larger blood vessels in the body have a name. For example, the main artery leaving the left side of the heart is called the *aorta*. Whenever the aorta divides to supply an organ, it takes a location name in order to assist anatomists to describe where they are in the body. An example of this would be the aortic division to supply the kidney with blood, called the *renal artery*. When blood leaves the kidney, the vessel is called the *renal vein* and this will rejoin the main vein, the *vena cava*.

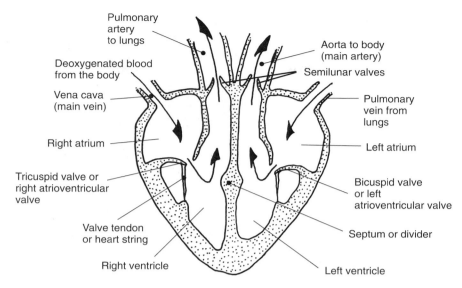

Fig. 3.2   The heart. Arrows indicate the direction of blood flow.

The heart

The heart lies between the two sides of the chest (the thorax), surrounded by the lungs, and is held in place by a structure called the *mediastinum* (Fig. 3.2). It is made up of a specialised muscle type which differs from others in three ways:

(1)   Made of branching muscle fibres connected to each other in the form of a network. This enables contractions to begin at one point in the heart and spread outwards in all directions.
(2)   Heart or cardiac muscle contracts and relaxes rhythmically in 'beats'. The rhythm is generated within the muscle itself and not by impulses from the nervous system.
(3)   Heart muscle does not get tired, despite continuous and rapid contractions over many years.

The heart consists of two pumps fused together, each having two chambers:

•   Right atrium and right ventricle
•   Left atrium and left ventricle

The right side of the heart is the less muscular side and pumps deoxygenated blood from the body to the lungs for reoxygenation. The left side of the heart is very muscular and is responsible for pumping oxygenated blood to the body (Fig. 3.3). The blood is under high pressure and this will ensure:

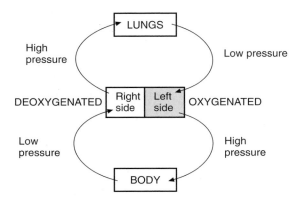

Fig. 3.3 The heart pump.

- Fast supply of materials to the cells and tissues
- Pushing of fluid from the circulation into the tissues

The heart is surrounded by a thick fibrous bag called the *pericardium*. Blood enters the heart from the body (systemic circulation) via the great veins, the *vena cava*, caudal and cranial vessels. The right atrium contracts to top up the right ventricle. When the right ventricle pumps, it pushes blood out through the pulmonary artery into the lungs (deoxygenated blood). After oxygenation of the blood in the lungs, the blood returns via the pulmonary veins to the left atrium. This contracts to pump the blood through to the left ventricle. The left ventricle is the most muscular chamber of the heart, in order to be able to pump blood around the rest of the body, via the *aorta*.

To stop blood flowing backwards (in the wrong direction), there are valves. On the *right* side of the heart there are the:

- Right atrioventricular valve, also called the tricuspid valve
- Semilunar valve, also called the pulmonary semilunar valve

and on the *left* side of the heart there are the:

- Left atrioventricular valve, also called the bicuspid or mitral valve
- Semilunar valve, also called aortic semilunar valve

At the base of the aorta, just above the semilunar valves, are the entrances to the left and right coronary arteries which supply the *myocardium* (the heart muscles). If these vessels narrow due to fatty deposits or cholesterol, this will reduce the blood flow to the heart muscle, causing lack of oxygen (*ischaemia*) when exercising. This in turn could lead to a heart attack, also called a coronary attack.

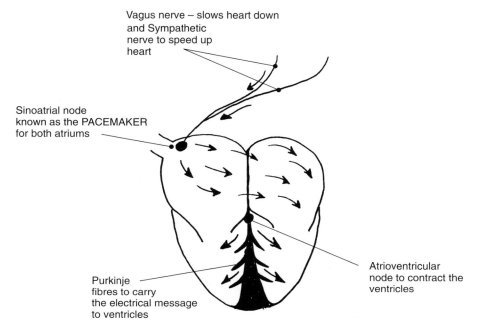

Fig. 3.4 Electrical activity during contraction of the heart (pumping). The rhythm for this is provided by the pacemaker.

Heart beat

Most muscles will contract as a result of impulses reaching them from nerves. The heart is a muscle which beats rhythmically from impulses within its structure. It has special fibres imbedded in the wall of the right atrium called the *sino-atrial node* or, more commonly, the *pacemaker* (Fig. 3.4). This area responds to chemicals like adrenaline or the nervous system command to increase the heart rate in situations of fear, flight or fight.

The electrical message from the pacemaker passes to the right and left atrium, causing them to contract in unison. The impulse then arrives at the atrioventricular node, before passing along special conducting tissue pathways called the *bundles of His*. These fibres lead to the smaller bundles of conducting tissues called *Purkinje fibres*, which cause contraction of the ventricles.

If the pacemaker region of the heart is malfunctioning, the heart rate may fall and not increase with exercise. An animal with this condition will have a slow heart rate with poor exercise tolerance and may faint.

Heart sounds

There are two sounds:

LUB – DUB

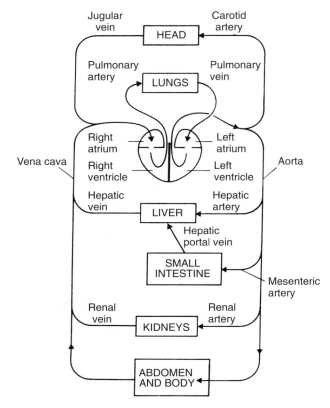

Fig. 3.5   Heart and circulation flow.

The first sound, Lub, is produced by the closure of the right and left atrioventricular valves, as the ventricles begin to contract.

When the valves at the base of the aorta and pulmonary artery (semilunar valves) snap shut at the end of the ventricle contraction, then the second sound, Dub, is produced.

If blood within the chest is flowing unevenly or turbulently, a murmur may be detected. This sounds like: Lub – woosh – Dub.

Respiratory system

Respiration is a term referring to the gaseous exchange between a living structure and its environment.

Structures through which oxygen and carbon dioxide (waste gas) must pass

External nares – nose
Turbinate bones – scroll-shaped tubes with epithelial lining in nasal chambers
Nasopharynx – back of the throat
Larynx – voice box
Trachea – open tube for passage of gases only
Bronchus – branching of the trachea to the two sides of the chest (thorax)
Bronchioles – further branching, getting smaller in diameter
Alveoli – air sacs
Blood capillaries of the pulmonary system
Tissue cells around the body

Characteristics of the respiratory surfaces

Below is a list of features common to all respiratory surfaces. They allow oxygen and carbon dioxide to be exchanged rapidly between an organism and the air which surrounds it.

- Respiratory surfaces have a large surface area to ensure maximum contact with the inhaled air. A mammal's respiratory surface consists of millions of tiny bubble-like air sacs called *alveoli*.
- All respiratory surfaces are moist. This is necessary because oxygen and carbon dioxide can only diffuse in a solution across a respiratory surface (alveoli to blood vessel).
- A respiratory surface is extremely thin, only one cell thick, so that diffusion can take place.
- The inside of a respiratory surface is in contact with a network of capillary blood vessels. This allows gas exchange to take place between the blood and gases.
- There is usually a mechanism which ensures that a respiratory surface is well ventilated, that it receives a steady flow of air. Breathing movements increase the rate of gas exchange by continually removing carbon dioxide and renewing supplies of oxygen to the tissue cells.

The role of breathing and the circulation

The respiratory and circulatory systems determine how much oxygen and carbon dioxide are present in the body at a given moment. If the amount of oxygen in the blood is low and carbon dioxide high, the body responds by increasing:

- The rate and depth of breathing – ventilation rate.
- The rate at which the heart beats – cardiac frequency.

- The diameter of the arterioles serving those structures that are short of oxygen – vasodilation.

The respiratory organs of mammals

The thoracic cavity, thorax or chest contains the:

- Heart
- Lungs
- Major blood vessels
- Lymph ducts
- Major nerves

The walls of the thorax are strengthened by the ribs (skeletal system) and caudally (towards the tail) consists of a sheet of muscle called the *diaphragm*. A system of passageways leads from the mouth and nostrils into the lungs and will now be described in more detail (Fig. 3.6).

The nasal passages

This is where air enters and is warmed to body temperature. The membranes covering the nasal passages also contain the organs responsible for the sense of smell. The walls and base of the nasal passages are lined with a carpet of microscopic hair-like structures called *cilia*. The cilia extend down the trachea to create a surface of moving hairs beating in an upward manner. They help to

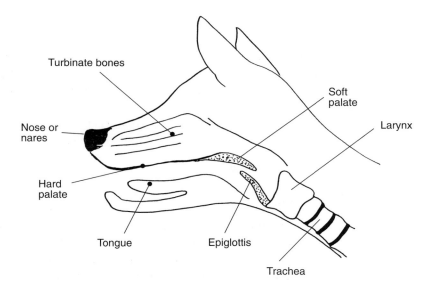

Fig. 3.6 Upper respiratory tract.

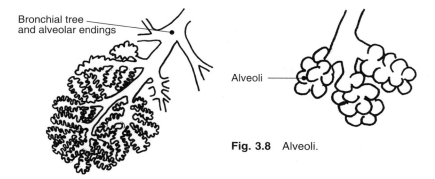

Bronchial tree
and alveolar endings

Alveoli

Fig. 3.8   Alveoli.

Fig. 3.7   Lung tissue.

expel mucus, which contains dust and micro-organisms which are held in this
thickened liquid.

Air is drawn out of the nasal passages into the pharynx at the back of the
mouth. From here, air is drawn into the trachea via the larynx and past the vocal
cords to activate the voice.

The bronchial tree

This is the main trunk of the branching trachea, as it supplies lung tissue on both
sides of the thorax. This then becomes the bronchi leading into each lobe of lung
tissue (Fig. 3.7). The bronchi will further divide many times to form a mass of fine
branches called the bronchioles.

The alveolar ducts

These are the tubes at the end of the bronchioles leading to the air sacs or alveoli
(Fig. 3.8). The alveoli are the respiratory surface of the lungs, giving lung tissue
its spongy appearance. The outer surface of the alveoli is covered by a dense
network of capillary blood vessels. All these capillaries originate from the pulmonary artery (deoxygenated blood) and drain into the pulmonary vein (oxygenated blood) to return to the left side of the heart, for pumping around the
body.

Gas exchange in the lungs

Blood entering the lungs is deoxygenated because the haemoglobin (red
pigment) in its red cells has given up all its oxygen to the body tissues.

The internal diameter of the lung capillaries is actually smaller than the diameter of the red cells which pass through them. The red cells therefore are squeezed
out of shape as they are forced through the lungs by blood pressure and the speed

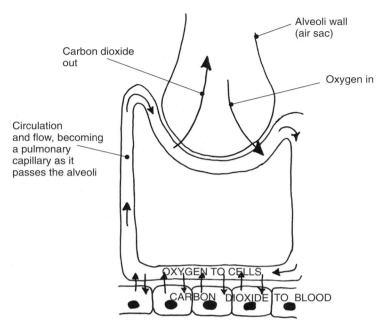

Fig. 3.9 Gas exchange between the alveoli and the blood and between the blood and body cells.

at which they move is considerably reduced by the resulting friction. This increases the rate of oxygen absorption in two ways:

(1) As the red cells squeeze through the narrow capillaries they expose more surface area to the capillary walls, through which oxygen is diffusing and absorbed.
(2) Their slow rate of progress increases the time available for oxygen to diffuse into the vessels and combine with haemoglobin.

The continuous removal of oxygen as fast as it diffuses into the lung capillaries and the continuous arrival of oxygen in the alveoli owing to breathing movements mean that there is always a higher concentration of oxygen molecules in the alveoli than in the blood. As a result of this, carbon dioxide is exchanged (Fig. 3.9).

Breathing – ventilation of the lungs

The thorax or pleural cavity is completely airtight and contains a partial vacuum. Its internal pressure is always less than the atmospheric pressure outside the body. The lungs are open to the atmosphere through the trachea and so there is always a higher pressure in the lungs than in the thorax or pleural cavity

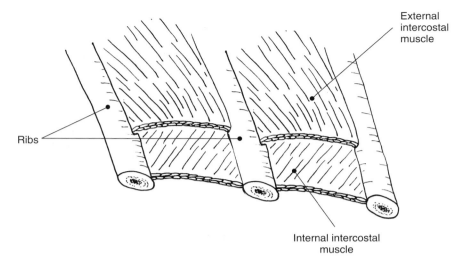

External
intercostal
muscle

Ribs

Internal intercostal
muscle

Fig. 3.10 Intercostal muscles and ribs for breathing.

which surrounds them. This pressure difference is extremely important for two reasons:

(1) The higher pressure in the lungs in relation to the pleural cavity around them stretches the thin elastic alveoli walls so that the lungs as a whole almost fill the thorax on inspiration.
(2) Since this pressure difference is maintained during breathing movements, when the thoracic cavity increases in size (inspiration), the lungs inflate to fill the extra space available.

At normal atmospheric pressure the above could not happen, hence the need for negative pressure in the thorax.

The muscles which bring about these volume changes are:

• *The diaphragm* – a dome-shaped sheet of muscle which separates the thorax from the abdomen.
• *The intercostal muscles* – both internal and external, that cross the gap between each rib and pull the ribs outwards on inspiration (Fig. 3.10).

Diaphragm

Immediately before inspiration, the diaphragm is dome-shaped and its muscle relaxed. Inspiration takes place when the diaphragm muscle contracts, making the muscle sheet a flatter shape.

Rib

At the same time, contraction occurs in the external intercostal muscles between each rib. This increases the size of the rib cage, leading to an increase in lung volume.

- *Inspiration* – the movement of the diaphragm and external intercostal muscles, causing the ribs to move visibly outwards.
- *Expiration* – or breathing out is when the diaphragm and external intercostal muscles relax. This reduces the size of the thorax and the ribs move inwards to the resting position.

Air can be forced out of the lungs by contraction of the internal intercostal muscles but expiration tends to be passive, simply allowing these structures to fall back into the resting position.

Respiration

The word 'respiration' is derived from the Latin *respirare* which means 'to breathe'. At first, this term referred to the breathing movements which cause air to be drawn into and pushed out of the lungs but now, when defined with strict accuracy, respiration means something entirely different.

The modern definition of respiration

The processes which lead to, and include, the chemical breakdown of materials to provide energy for life. These processes occur inside the living cells of every type of organism and cause the release of energy from food which is essential for life.

Cells cannot use energy as soon as it is released from respiration. This energy is first used to build up a temporary energy store, which takes the form of a chemical called *adenosine triphosphate* or ATP for short. Think of ATP as 'packets' of energy, used to transfer energy from the chemical reactions which release it to the body processes which use it. Respiration fills these ATP packets with energy and they are 'emptied' when energy is needed anywhere in the body.

There are four main advantages to the ATP energy transfer system.

(1) ATP takes up some energy which would otherwise be lost as heat during the breakdown of glucose by respiratory enzymes.
(2) Energy is released from ATP the instant it is required without cells having to go through the many different reactions of respiration, allowing for sudden bursts of energy.
(3) ATP delivers energy in precise amounts.

(4)   Energy can be delivered from ATP to other chemicals without energy loss; for example, from sources of sugars, fats or proteins.

The release of energy at the cellular level is known as the *Krebs cycle*.

Digestive system

An animal is able to make full use of the food it eats after the following events have taken place, through the digestive tract (Fig. 3.11).

- Food is first torn up into pieces small enough to swallow (*mastication*).
- Food enters the alimentary canal mixed with digestive enzymes to further break down the food into simple water-soluble chemicals – the process of *digestion*. It takes place outside the cells of the body.
- The soluble food then passes through the walls of the gut into the bloodstream. This is called *absorption*.
- Blood then transports the digested, soluble food to all parts of the body. The food enters cells and is transformed into substances which take part in the body's metabolism. This is called *assimilation*.
- Any solid substances in food which cannot be digested, like fibres, are expelled from the body as faecal matter or faeces.

Foods

Most foods which animals eat cannot be used by their bodies in the original form for two main reasons:

(1)   Most foods are insoluble and so cannot pass through cell membranes into cells.
(2)   Most foods are chemically different from the substances that make up body tissues. They must therefore be processed before the body can use them by the use of enzymes.

Digestive enzymes

All enzymes, whether digestive or belonging to another body system, are *catalysts*. They speed up chemical reactions which would otherwise proceed very slowly. Digestive enzymes are only one example of the many types of enzymes which exist in living animals. The reactions which these enzymes speed up involve splitting complicated molecules into simpler ones.

It is thought that the enzyme combines briefly with molecules of food and while in this state the food undergoes a rapid chemical change in which its molecules are split apart into chemically simpler substances. These substances separate from the enzyme, leaving it immediately available for another identical reaction.

Enzymes are not used up in the reactions which they control but are used countless times in rapid succession.

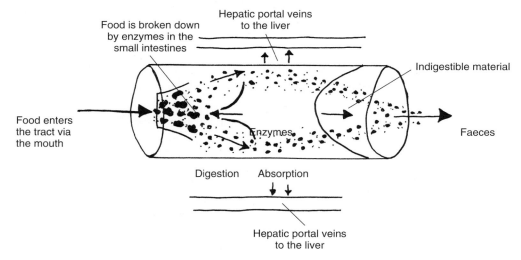

Fig. 3.11   Digestive tract – events.

Comparative digestive anatomy

The digestive tract or alimentary canal is simply a continuous tube, with different regions along its length performing different functions.

Anatomically, different species of mammals are grouped according to their digestive anatomy (Figs 3.12 and 3.13).

- Ruminants or polygastric animals (cattle and sheep)
- Simple-stomached animals (e.g. dog, cat and humans)
- Avian (all birds)
- Monogastric herbivores (the horse)

Other definitions may refer to the type of food eaten.

- Carnivores – meat eating
- Omnivores – eat both meat and vegetable matter
- Herbivores – grass eating
- Grainivores – grain eating

The control of digestion of food is both voluntary and involuntary.

- Voluntary
  - (a)   Ingestion – placing in mouth
  - (b)   Chewing

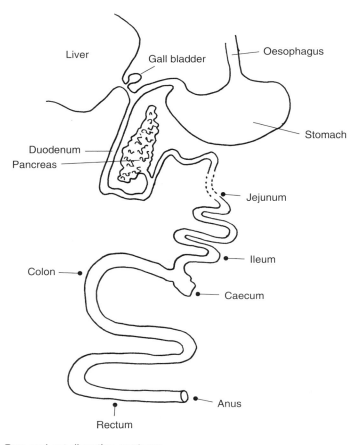

Fig. 3.12   Dog and cat digestive anatomy.

(c)   Swallowing (deglutition)
(d)   Control of anal sphincter – the muscle controlling the opening and closing of the anus
- Involuntary
  (a)   Opening and closing of sphincters
  (b)   Peristaltic movement (a ripple or wave of muscle) squeezing the food through the gut
  (c)   Release of digestive enzymes

Digestive tract of dog and cat

- Mouth
- Pharynx
- Oesophagus
- Stomach

The stomach

The oesophagus enters the stomach via a ring of muscle called the *cardiac sphincter*, a structure which adapts itself to the quantity of food eaten. Some digestion occurs here and the stomach acts as a temporary reservoir. The gastric juices, which contain enzymes and hydrochloric acid, start breaking up the food. The well-mixed and partially digested food, now called *chyme*, is now moved through the sphincter at the stomach exit, called the *pylorus*, and on to the first section of the small intestine.

The small intestines

So called because of their narrow bore, not their length. Enzyme digestion is completed in the small intestines.

- Protein is converted to amino acids
- Fat is converted to fatty acids
- Carbohydrates are converted to simple sugars

The chyme is mixed with more enzymes in the first section of the small intestines, the *duodenum*. Some will originate from the duodenum, others from the *pancreas* (its *exocrine* function). The liver also secretes a digestive fluid into the duodenum via the gall bladder; this fluid is ducted into the small intestine to reduce the size of fatty acid molecules and is called *bile*. Bile helps by emulsifying fats and will neutralise the acid fluids from the stomach because it is alkaline.

The second section of the small intestines, called the *jejunum*, continues the mixing and exposing of the chyme to the fluids that reduce it sufficiently for absorption.

The third section of the small intestines is the *ileum*, where the final absorption is completed.

Digestion and absorption are improved by the enormous surface area in the small intestine. Features of this area include:

- The great length of the intestines
- The presence of folds of tissue, increasing the surface area
- The arrangement of finger-like projections called *villi*
- The great number of these villi on the surface of the small intestine, particularly in the final area, the ileum, for maximum absorption

Absorption. This takes place via the villi (Fig. 3.18). They contain smooth muscle which allows them to contract and expand. This action brings them into contact with the newly digested food. Simple sugars (mainly glucose) and amino acids

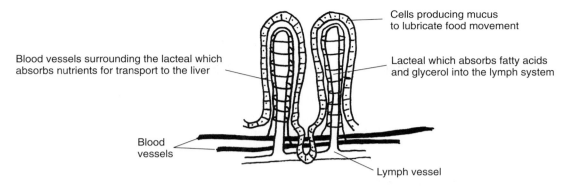

Cells producing mucus
to lubricate food movement

Blood vessels surrounding the lacteal which
absorbs nutrients for transport to the liver

Lacteal which absorbs fatty acids
and glycerol into the lymph system

Blood
vessels

Lymph vessel

Fig. 3.18   The villi.

are absorbed, by a combination of diffusion and active transport, across the epithelial lining of the villi into the waiting capillaries beneath. These capillaries drain into the hepatic portal vein which leads to the liver.

Fat is dealt with differently. The fatty acids and glycerol are absorbed into the columnar epithelial cells lining the villi and are pushed into the lymph vessels of the villi as a white emulsion of tiny globules of fat. These globules give the lymph vessels a milky appearance, for which they are known as *lacteals*. The lymph system opens finally into the veins in the thorax and empties via the thoracic duct into the vena cava near the heart.

Salts, vitamins and water are also absorbed in the small intestine.

The large intestines

This section of intestines is a wider tube and contains no villi. Food materials which are of no value or cannot be broken down to absorbable size are passed from the small to the large intestine through the *ileocaecal valve*. The large intestine in the dog and cat is relatively short in length. Its main purpose is to absorb salt and water. The walls of the colon (large intestine) are much folded for this purpose. By the time materials reach the rectum, indigestible food is in a semi-solid condition ready to be voided through the anus as faeces.

The first part of the large intestines is called the *caecum*. It is a blind-ended sac which has no function in carnivores but is enlarged in herbivores as a site of bacterial breakdown of vegetable food matter.

The colon is divided into three sections:

- Ascending
- Transverse
- Descending

The colon terminates in the rectum area, where waste products are held before excretion as faecal material.

The last part of the tract is closed by sphincter muscles and is known as the anal canal, over which the animal has control via skeletal muscle (voluntary muscle). Defecation involves relaxation of the anal sphincter but diarrhoea or illness may override this control. Diarrhoea is defined as the frequent evacuation of watery faeces. If defecation is delayed too long, constipation may result.

Consistent with its functions of water absorption and faecal movement, the large intestine is lined with a mucus-secreting surface. This assists in the movement of materials by a lubricating action. The mucus prevents the total drying out of the faeces, which might then damage the lining.

Brief summary of digestion and absorption of the main food constituents

- *Proteins* – come from muscle meat, egg or vegetable proteins like soya bean. These are broken down in the stomach and small intestines to become amino acids and absorbed into the bloodstream for transport to the liver, where they are processed.
- *Carbohydrates* – are found as cereals like biscuit potatoes or pasta. They are broken down into simple sugars (*glucose*) and absorbed into the bloodstream for transport to the liver where they may be stored as *glycogen*. When required by the body for energy, glycogen can be turned back into glucose.
- *Fats* – are found as animal fat or vegetable oils and are broken down into fatty acids and glycerols by bile and enzymes in the small intestines. Most will enter the lacteals in the villi to travel via the lymph system, finally reaching the bloodstream for use or storage.

Liver and pancreas

The liver is the largest organ of the body, situated immediately caudal to the diaphragm in the abdomen. About 75% of the liver's blood supply comes from the hepatic portal system of vessels (Fig. 3.19). This ensures that the products of digestion are absorbed into the bloodstream and travel to the liver for processing, before moving on either to storage or to be used in another way. The remaining 25% of blood to the liver arrives via the hepatic artery.

The special cells that make up the liver are called *hepatocytes*. The liver is a very complex chemical factory which produces materials for use within the body from the products of digestion which come directly to it from the gut.

Functions of the liver

It is thought that the liver performs over 500 functions. The main functions are as follows:

- Regulation of sugar which has four possible fates:
  (1)   used as energy source (Krebs cycle)

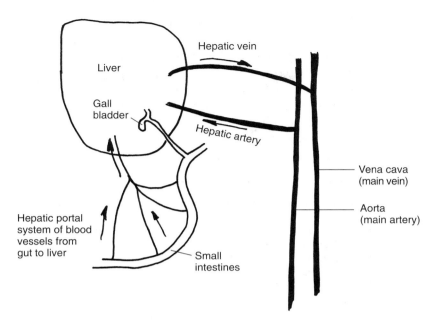

Fig. 3.19 Blood supply to the liver.

(2)   stored as glycogen in the liver
(3)   converted to fat and stored around the body
(4)   passed directly into the circulation
- Regulation of lipids (fats)
- Regulation of amino acids and proteins
- Heat production
- Bile production
- Formation of cholesterol
- Elimination of sex hormones
- Storage and filtration of blood
- Elimination of haemoglobin from exhausted red blood cells
- Formation of urea to be passed on to the kidneys for removal from the body
- Creation of plasma proteins (synthesis)
- Storage of vitamins A, D and B_{12} and minerals like iron and copper

The pancreas

The pancreas is a large grey-pink gland, which lies in the abdomen close to the stomach and the duodenum section of the small intestine. It is made up of two parts which are joined together, giving the pancreas its boomerang shape.

There are two types of tissue present within the gland and these have very different functions.

- *Exocrine tissue* – which produces digestive enzymes
- *Endocrine tissue* – which produces hormones like insulin to help in controlling sugar in the body.

Urinary system

This system has several functions but its main one is that of excretion and removal of waste products from the body. Wastes are toxic if allowed to accumulate so this removal of harmful materials, which are the end products of metabolism, is essential and continuous.

> **Functions include:**
>
> - loss or conservation of body water
> - excretion of unwanted substances or those in excess to requirements
> - storage of products before their removal from the body
> - endocrine organ producing hormones.

The mammalian urinary tract consists of:

- Two kidneys
- Two ureters
- One bladder
- One urethra

The kidneys

These are bean shaped and situated one on each side of the abdomen (Fig. 3.20). Each contains specialised cells which filter out materials which must be removed from the body and conserve those which the body needs. These cells are called the *nephrons*, from which we get the term *nephritis*, meaning inflammation of the kidney nephron cells.

The blood supply to the kidneys is via the renal artery directly from the aorta and drains away from the kidney via the renal vein directly into the vena cava.

The nephron

This is the special cell of the urinary system. The structure is as follows (Fig. 3.21):

- *Glomerulus* – a network or knot of artery from branches of the renal artery in the cortex section of the kidney.

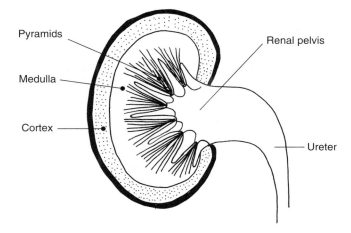

Fig. 3.20   The kidney.

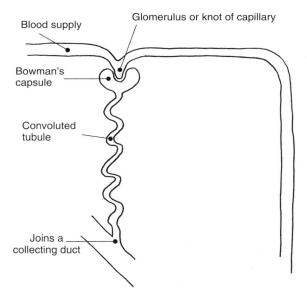

Fig. 3.21   The nephron.

- *Bowman's capsule* – the cup-shaped part of the nephron, at the start of the tubule. It is into this that the glomerulus fits and contacts, resulting in the start of blood filtration and the removal of urea and other nitrogenous wastes.
- *Proximal tubule* – the start of the long tube through which the filtered substances will pass.
- *Loop of Henle and distal tubule* – this is where, on instruction from hormones, the nephron conserves water, salts and sugars or, if the body has an excess, it is instructed to add the excess to the forming urine for removal from the body.

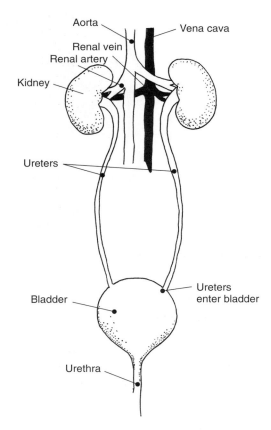

Fig. 3.22 The urinary system.

The distal tubule joins a collecting duct which directs the urine to the pelvis region of the kidney, where all nephrons drain, then along the ureter to the bladder for temporary storage. When the bladder is full, the animal receives this information from the brain and relaxes the sphincter muscle from the bladder to the urethra and the outside (Fig. 3.22). The act of passing urine is called *micturition*.

Nervous system

The nervous system provides the quickest means of communication within the body. Information is received both from outside the animal (the environment) and from inside the animal's body. The response to information received has to be co-ordinated in order for the body systems to unite in their response, to produce the desired effect.

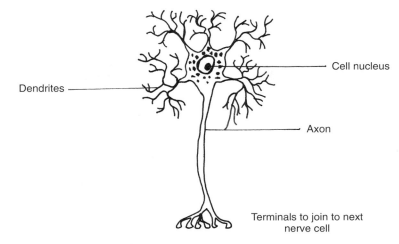

Dendrites

Cell nucleus

Axon

Terminals to join to next nerve cell

Fig. 3.23 Nerve cell – the neurone.

Messages to the body are carried in two ways:

(1) *Electrical* – these are impulses which travel along the nerves and give fast response to a situation or stimulus (nervous system). The electrical messages stimulate movement of muscles:
    (a) cardiac – the heart
    (b) skeletal – bones and joints
    (c) involuntary – organs and tissues.
(2) *Chemical* – these are hormones which, once released into the bloodstream, will travel more slowly to their target organ. The body response is seen after a period of time (endocrine system).

Body co-ordination by nervous system tissue is conducted by the nerve cells, the *neurones* (Fig. 3.23), together with various forms of supporting tissue in which they are embedded. These cells are the basic functional unit of the nervous system and are found in bundles, called *nerves*.

There are four types of neurone.

(1) *Sensory* – those attached to the senses, like sight, hearing, taste, smell and touch. These carry messages about information outside the body to the brain.
(2) *Relay* – information or messages between neurones.
(3) *Motor* – these link up to relay neurones and with muscle or gland cells in order to deliver messages from the central nervous system (brain and spinal cord) to initiate an action. This may be the release of more hormone or the movement of a muscle.

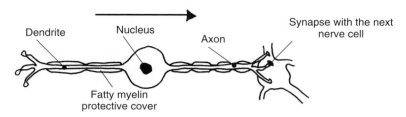

Fig. 3.24   Nerve cell and direction of electrical impulse.

(4)   *Network* – these link the cell branches in order to keep the information and action by the brain and spinal cord networked like a computer.

The shape of the nerve cell will vary to suit the tissue into which it links but the basic components remain the same.

- A cell body containing the nucleus.
- Cell processes which lead to and from the cell body (Fig. 3.24):
  (a)   the *axon* – which carries the impulses away from the cell body
  (b)   the *dendrite* – which carries impulses towards the cell body.

The property of a nerve cell is that its cell membrane is electrically charged by the action of *ions* (salts or electrolytes) such as potassium or sodium. Although the voltage carried is small, when discharged along the length of nerves, it allows the system to act as a high-speed electrical signalling system. After the signal, the membrane is recharged and returns to a resting position, awaiting the next signal.

The junction between two or more neurones is called a *synapse* (Fig. 3.25). Electrical impulses cannot pass across this gap, so communication is dependent upon a chemical transmitter substance – a *neurotransmitter*. This substance will connect two neurones for less than one millisecond, allowing the impulse to pass on. The chemical is then destroyed by another substance and recreated again before each future impulse.

Reflex action or arc (Fig. 3.26)

This refers to an automatic and very rapid response to a potentially harmful stimulus which is usually external to the body. It is a survival response.

The structural basis of reflex action is the *reflex arc*, which represents the series of units of nerve tissue through which impulses have to pass in order to bring about a reflex response. The sensory tissues receiving the information are called *receptors* and may be scattered sensory cells in the skin or special sense receptors like the eye or ear. Their stimulation results in impulses being generated in

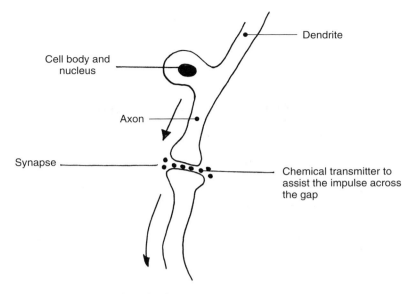

Fig. 3.25   A synapse – the junction between two or more neurones.

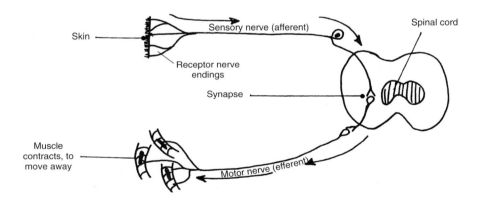

Fig. 3.26   Reflex arc.

sensory (*afferent*) neurones located in the peripheral nerves (on or near the body surface). These afferent neurones take the impulse to the central nervous system (only to the spinal cord) where a connection nerve in the cord connects to a motor (*efferent*) neurone. This will take the impulse or message to an effector tissue like a gland or to a muscle for the desired effect – survival.

The common example used is touching a hot surface, when the reflex arc ensures that the animal suffers minimal harm as the foot is speedily withdrawn from the danger.

Central nervous system

Made up of the brain and spinal cord.

The brain

The general function of the brain is to co-ordinate the body's activities. It receives all sensory information and processes it for:

- Immediate use – reflex arc.
- Later use – storing it in memory, passing orders via neurones and hormones, constantly monitoring the internal body systems for any change.

The brain is divided into three parts (Fig. 3.27).

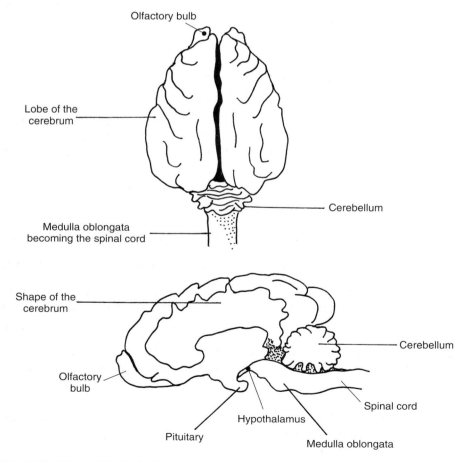

Fig. 3.27 Parts of the brain, from two views.

(1) *Forebrain* – cerebrum, divided into two areas called the cerebral hemispheres (including the hypothalamus), involved with voluntary movement and the senses.
(2) *Midbrain* – involved with sight, hearing, muscle control and body position.
(3) *Hindbrain* – the cerebellum, the pons and the medulla oblongata. Involved with complicated movements of the body, control of the circulation and respiration and awareness of surroundings.

The spinal cord

The cord extends from the base of the skull to the lumbar/sacral region of the spine, over the pelvis. It is a continuation of the hindbrain and medulla oblongata. The cord is protected by the *vertebrae* and the *meninges*. The canal, which runs through each vertebra, houses the spinal cord.

The cord divides into many branching spinal nerves. This continues first inside the vertebrae, then on the outside of the coccygeal vertebrae as the *cauda equina* (resembling a horse's tail), to supply motor and sensory nerves to the tip of the animal's tail.

Protection of the brain and spinal cord

- *Bones* – skull and bones of the spine.
- *Meninges* – the three membranes, in turn separated by the cerebrospinal fluid.
- *Blood–brain barrier* – a mechanism located in a continuous layer of endothelial cells which allows only useful substances to enter the brain.

Meninges

The three protective membranes covering the brain and spinal cord

- *Dura mater* – the tough outer membrane, in contact with the bone of the skull and the vertebrae.
- *Arachnoid* – a fine network of collagen and elastic fibres, next to the dura mater.
- *Pia mater* – the membrane in contact with the brain and spinal cord tissue surface.

Peripheral nervous system

Voluntary nervous system

- Paired spinal nerves containing both sensory and motor fibres, forming a mixed spinal nerve.
- Twelve cranial nerves. These are mixed nerves and can contain motor and sensory, voluntary and autonomic fibres (Table 3.2).

Table 3.2 The 12 cranial nerves.

Number	Name	Type	Function
I	Olfactory	Sensory	Smell
II	Optic	Sensory	Vision, pupil light response
III	Oculomotor	Motor	Eye movement, pupil constriction
IV	Trochlear	Motor	Eye movement
V	Trigeminal	Mixed	Mastication, touch and pain receptors
VI	Abducens	Motor	Eye movement
VII	Facial	Mixed	Salivation, facial expression, taste
VIII	Auditory/ vestibulocochlear	Sensory	Hearing, balance
IX	Glossopharyngeal	Mixed	Taste, laryngeal muscles
X	Vagus	Mixed	Vocalisation, swallowing Decrease in heart rate Abdominal organs
XI	Accessory	Motor	Head movement
XII	Hypoglossal	Motor	Tongue movement

Involuntary or autonomic nervous system

- Sympathetic nervous system
- Parasympathetic nervous system

The involuntary or autonomic nervous system is not under conscious control and is involved with the regulation of body functions. It is divided into two parts, distinguished by their function and by the chemical transmitters (neurotransmitters) used at the synapse between nerve cells.

Sympathetic system	**Parasympathetic system**
Chemical – adrenaline	Chemical – cholinesterase
Prepares body for fight, fright and flight	Assists in day-to-day function of the body
Inhibits salivation	Stimulates salivation
Increases heart rate	Decreases heart rate back to normal
Increases respiratory rate	Decreases respiratory rate

Endocrine system

This is made up of a system of ductless glands which are sites for the production of hormones (Fig. 3.28). The hormones are discharged directly into the blood for circulation to the target organ or tissue. Hormones are sometimes referred to as chemical messengers.

Protection of the eyes

- Cavities in the skull called the *orbits* protect the eye ball with a bone and cartilage ring.
- The transparent, self-repairing skin on the eye called the conjunctiva.
- Tears keep the eyes moist; a stream of liquid from the tear glands is wiped across the eye by blinking and prevents the tissues from becoming too dry.
- The blink reflex to guard against dust and other objects which might enter the eye socket.

Nourishment and support tissues of the eye

The eye receives oxygen via blood vessels which enter with the optic nerve, at the back of the eye. These vessels spread out through the *choroid layer* and over the surface of the *retina*.

The *cornea* and *lens* obtain oxygen and food by diffusion from vessels in the liquid in the front chamber of the eye – the *aqueous humour*.

Vitreous humour is a jelly in the back cavity of the eye which helps to maintain the shape of the eye.

The *iris* is the coloured part of the eye and has a round hole in its centre called the *pupil*. The iris consists of muscles which radiate out and contract to enlarge the size of the pupil and circular muscles, which make it smaller in size. The iris regulates the amount of light reaching the retina.

The lens consists of layers of transparent material arranged like the skins of an onion, which are enclosed in an elastic outer membrane. These are held in place by *suspensory ligaments*, which in turn are attached to a ring of muscle called the *ciliary muscle*.

The retina is covered with light-sensitive receptors called *rods and cones* (due to their shape). These are buried under nerve fibres and a layer of blood capillaries which conduct the impulses to the brain. These layers are absent from the area where the clearest image is formed, the *fovea*. This area is directly opposite the lens and is the most sensitive part of the eye for colour vision.

The retina contains an area called the *blind spot* (Fig. 3.30). It consists of blood

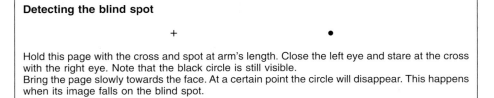

Detecting the blind spot

Hold this page with the cross and spot at arm's length. Close the left eye and stare at the cross with the right eye. Note that the black circle is still visible.
Bring the page slowly towards the face. At a certain point the circle will disappear. This happens when its image falls on the blind spot.

Fig. 3.30   Detecting the eye's blind spot.

vessels and nerve fibres leading to the optic nerve. Due to these tissues this area is completely insensitive to light.

The ear

The anatomy of the ear is shown in Fig. 3.31. Functions are:

*   Hearing
*   Detecting change in body position
*   Balance

The ear is divided into three sections:

(1)   *Outer* – for sound gathering.
(2)   *Middle* – transmits vibrations to the oval window of the inner ear.
(3)   *Inner* – receives the sound waves, passes them to the nerve that connects to the brain for conversion into hearing.

Outer ear

This is made up of the earflap or *pinna* and the canal. The shape of the canal will vary between species and breeds. This part of the ear collects sound waves and

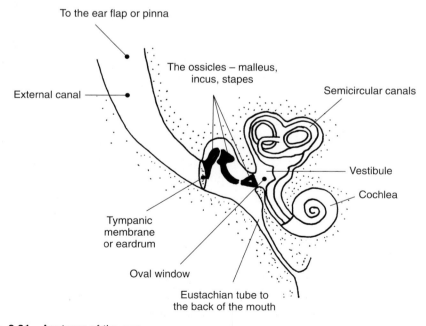

Fig. 3.31   Anatomy of the ear.

directs them into the canal, which is lined with modified sebaceous glands. These glands produce wax, as a protective layer. The canal leads to the eardrum or *tympanic membrane*.

Middle ear

This lies beyond the eardrum in the tympanic cavity, which is made of bone, on the ventral surface of the skull. The cavity contains three small bones called *ossicles*.

* *Malleus* – known as the hammer (contacts the eardrum)
* *Incus* – known as the anvil
* *Stapes* – known as the stirrup (contacts the oval window)

Vibrations of the eardrum (tympanic membrane) are transmitted by these bones to the *oval window*, which is the junction between the middle and inner ear.

The link between the middle ear and the throat/pharynx is the *auditory tube* (*Eustachian tube*). This tube allows air pressure to be equalised on either side of the eardrum.

Inner ear

This is situated in the temporal bone of the skull. It is here that sound vibrations are converted into nervous impulses and the inner ear is also involved in maintaining balance.

This area consists of a closed system of delicate tubes, called the *membranous labyrinth*, which contains a fluid caued *endolymph*. The labyrinth is itself bathed in a separate fluid, the *perilymph*.

The labyrinth is made up of:

* The *vestibule* – a sac-like structure.
* The *semicircular canals* – these are three loops at right angles to each other. They respond to movement of the endolymph, the angle of the head and changes in body position.
* The *cochlea* – a snail-shaped structure responsible for converting sound waves into nerve impulses which are converted in the brain to hearing.

Other senses

Smell or olfaction is important for the selection of food and scenting other animals. Olfactory membranes can also receive stimuli from the mouth so as a result, taste is sometimes actually smell.

Taste or gustation arises from taste cells contained in the mucous membranes

of the mouth and on the base of the tongue. Taste and smell will stimulate salivation and the digestive tract in readiness for food to be swallowed.

Jacobson's organ, or the vomeronasal organ, supplements the sense of smell in
receiving pheromone information about other animals. It is involved in the location of an animal on heat for reproductive purposes.

Skin or integument

The anatomy of the skin is shown in Fig. 3.32.

Function

- *Protection* – from the external environment and the controlled internal environment of the body, actively preventing:
  (a)   water loss
  (b)   absorption of toxic or harmful substances
  (c)   entry of disease-producing micro-organisms (*pathogens*).
- *Production* – of vitamin D which is required for the absorption of calcium
  from the intestines.
- *Sense organ* – receptor nerves throughout the skin's surface respond to:
  (a)   touch
  (b)   temperature
  (c)   pressure
  (d)   pain.

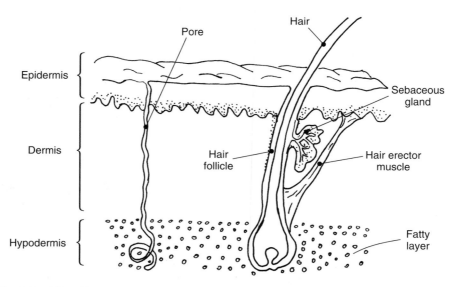

Fig. 3.32   The skin.

- *Storage* – of fat as adipose tissue. This is a body energy store and acts as an insulation layer to help maintain body temperature in cold weather.
- *Temperature control*
  - (a) For heat loss:
    - – vasodilation of surface blood vessels (widening of the vessel wall)
    - – sweating.
  - (b) For heat gain:
    - – vasoconstriction of blood vessels (narrowing of the vessel wall)
    - – erection of surface hair/coat/feathers to trap a layer of air for insulation
    - – a fat layer under the skin (*subcutaneous layer*).
- *Scent gland* – for communication with other animals for reproductive purposes (production of pheromones) or territorial purposes (use of the anal glands on either side of the anus).

Structure

- *Epidermis* – is the outer layer, which is hard and dry and contains no blood vessels. This layer continually looses dead cells.
- *Dermis* – is the layer below the epidermis and is a type of connective tissue containing nerves, blood vessels, glands and hair roots.
- *Hypodermis* – is the innermost layer of the skin.

Hair

This covers most of an animal's surface area. It is made of *keratin* (a protein made by the body) and pigments for colour. It grows from the hair *follicle* and attached to the deepest section of the hair is the smooth (involuntary) muscle called the *erector pili* muscle which is responsible for moving the hair upright.

Sweat glands

Sweat or sebaceous glands produce *sebum* which will include a pheromone. Other very specialised glands in the skin include mammary glands for milk production and anal glands for scenting territory.

Skeleton

The anatomy of the skeleton is shown in Fig. 3.33a. Figs 3.33b and c show the differences between dog and cat skeletons.

The skeleton is divided into three parts:

(1) *Axial* – skull, vertebral column (spine), ribs and sternum.
(2) *Appendicular* – the fore and hind limbs.
(3) *Splanchnic* – bones that develop in tissues, such as the os penis and fabellae.

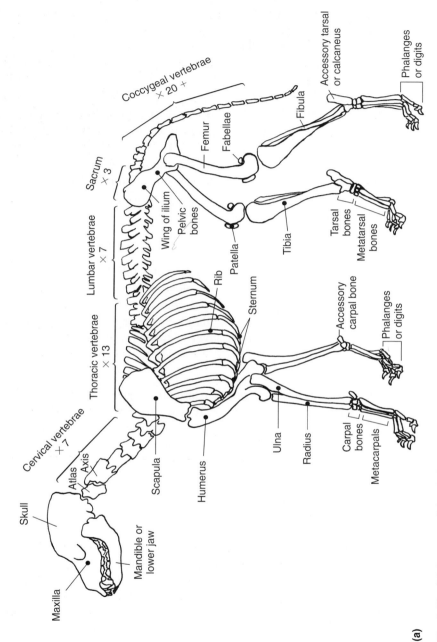

Fig. 3.33 (a) Anatomy of the skeleton.

Chapter 6
Animal Welfare

Welfare status

Welfare has many different aspects. There is no simple scale of expression and the problems are many and diverse in their nature. One method of expressing this diversity is known as 'The Five Freedoms', which relate particularly to UK farm animal welfare and suggest that the following are essential for quality of life:

- Freedom from hunger and thirst
- Freedom to express normal behaviour
- Freedom from discomfort
- Freedom from pain, injury and disease
- Freedom from fear or distress

Although initially set out to provide a useful framework for farm animal welfare and guidance, the above is also a suggested framework for companion animals.

Welfare terms

Animal welfare – refers to an animal's:

- quality of life
- conditions
- treatment

It is a concept that involves values as well as information. These values consider the ways in which humans continue to use animals and whether or not this 'use' constitutes animal abuse.

Animal rights – refers to animal use in industries, recreation and other practices as cruel, unethical and outdated, and calls for their abolition.

Conservation – refers to the consideration of the needs of one species, above another, of animals in the wild; the promotion of human understanding and education of animal habitats, affinity with certain species and the direct effect human activity can have on their welfare and survival.

Legislation

This covers both laws and regulations specific to the welfare of an animal or animal collection. These are combined with the professional working standards set by carers of animals.

Laws are guidelines and are changing all the time. It is therefore the responsibility of all animal carers to:

- Maintain a practical working knowledge of the law relating to animals
- Always work within that law

Legislation in the UK refers to both Acts of Parliament and Regulations.

- *Laws* (statutes) – are created by Parliament. Presented as draft legislation in the form of a bill, they are debated initially in the House of Commons and the House of Lords. They are each then considered by a specifically formed parliamentary committee, before finally receiving the Queen's signature to become law and being placed on the Statute Book as an Act of Parliament.
- *Regulations* (orders) – these detail the technical implications of laws. The relevant government minister adds regulations to the legislation. This information is a supplement to existing law and must have the approval of Parliament.

Welfare codes must also have parliamentary approval. Failure to comply with the provisions of a code is not in itself an offence, but could be used in evidence if prosecuted.

In addition to the above, we must abide by standards set by the European Union (EU) which have been incorporated into, and take precedence over, UK law.

Animal welfare legislation aims to:

- Balance concern for ethics and morality
- Balance financial and practical working considerations
- Ensure public health and safety
- State housing and transport requirements
- Maintain animal health
- Control licensing

Areas of the law relating to animal concerns in the UK are:

(1) Protection of the public laws
(2) Welfare laws to cover:
 – keeping of animals for commercial reasons
 – cruelty laws

(3)   Animal collection laws
(4)   Welfare of wild animals laws

Protection of the public laws

- Animal Health Act 1981
- Pet Travel Scheme
- Dangerous Dogs Acts 1991, 1997
- Guard Dogs Act 1975
- Animals Act 1971
- Dogs (Fouling of Land) Act 1996

Animal Health Act 1981 and rabies legislation

This Act gives powers for dealing with a rabies suspect and any contacts, under the Rabies (Control) Order 1974. In addition, the Animal Health Act 1981 allows government officers to slaughter affected or suspected animals and those that have been exposed to the infection. The orders and regulations covered by the Rabies (Control) Order 1974 include:

- Reporting of rabies to the Department for Environment, Food and Rural Affairs (DEFRA), local authority inspector or police
- Declaration of the infected place where a suspected animal is identified
- Slaughter of a suspected animal by a veterinary inspector
- Declaration of an 'infected area' around the place where the suspect animal was located, in order to control an outbreak of suspected rabies. This can also control movement, detention or destruction of animals not properly controlled, compulsory vaccination, prevention of any animal gatherings, e.g. dog shows, or any activity that might cause wildlife to move excessively through their environment.

The Rabies (Importation of Dogs, Cats and Other Mammals) Order 1974 (as amended) also provides the Secretary of State with the power to extend the quarantine period of any animal detained at a quarantine premises if:

(1)   An outbreak of rabies occurs at a quarantine premises
(2)   An animal in quarantine is suspected of being infected by rabies

The Rabies (Control) Order 1974 also applies to suspected cases in quarantine premises. Movement of animals into and out of the premises would stop, including those animals covered by the requirements of the Pet Travel Scheme.

Pet Travel Scheme

The Pet Travel Scheme, known as PETS, is the system that allows pet animals from certain countries to enter the UK without going into quarantine, as long as they comply with the rules under the scheme. It also allows pet owners from the UK to take and return with their pets having visited EU countries and some non-EU (listed) qualifying countries.

Animals from unlisted countries must spend 6 months in quarantine on arrival in the UK.

Animals returning to the UK from listed or EU countries under the PETS scheme must have followed a list of procedures to comply with the scheme. The procedures must be undertaken in the following order:

(1) The pet animal must be microchipped in order for it to be identified
(2) It must be vaccinated against rabies
(3) It must have a blood test to ensure that the vaccine has given it a satisfactory level of protection against rabies
(4) The owner must organise the documentation:
    – for an EU country an EU pet passport is required
    – for a non-EU country it is necessary to obtain an official third-country veterinary certificate (Gibraltar and Switzerland also issue passports)
(5) Before re-entry to the UK, the pet animal must be treated against ticks and tapeworms 24–48 hours before it is checked in with an approved transport company for its journey into the UK
(6) Arrangements must be made for the pet animal to travel with an approved transport company on an authorised route

For details of countries taking part in this scheme and the latest information, always check the DEFRA website.

There is a 6-month rule for entry or re-entry to the UK, which states that a dog or cat may not enter the UK under PETS until six calendar months have passed from the date that a blood sample was taken by a veterinary surgeon with satisfactory test results. Once the veterinary surgeon has issued the PETS documentation and that 6-month period has passed, the PETS documentation is valid for the named animal to enter the UK.

The scheme applies to:

• Pet dogs (to include assistance dogs) and cats
• Ferrets
• Pet rabbits and other rodents

Enforcing the new system:

• Pre-entry checks carried out by train operators, ferry companies and airlines
• Random spot checks on animals arriving in the UK by DEFRA and official carriers

Dangerous Dogs Acts 1991, 1997

After an increase in the number of attacks on people by dogs in the 1980s and 1990s, some fatal, the government introduced laws making it more difficult to own and import into the UK the following breeds of dog:

- American pit bull terrier
- Japanese tosa
- Dogo Argentino
- Fila Braziliero

The Act states that the rules for ownership of a dangerous named breed of dog are as follows:

- Notify the police of ownership
- Obtain a certificate of exemption from the police, which is issued when the dog has been neutered and identified with a microchip or other permanent method
- The dog must be covered by third-party liability insurance
- In public places, the dog must always be muzzled and on a lead
- The dog must be in the company of a person over 16 years of age
- It is an offence to sell, exchange or abandon the dog
- It is an offence to breed from these dogs

Any dog dangerously out of control and a risk to the general public comes under the remit of this Act. The person in charge of a dog that has inflicted injury could be prosecuted and face an unlimited fine or prison sentence.

Guard Dogs Act 1974

This Act ensures the safe use and control of dogs that guard property or sites, in a manner that does not put the general public at risk. A notice must be on display to inform the public that a dog is in use and the dog must only be off the lead if accompanied by a handler.

Animals Act 1971

This Act covers liability for damage that has been caused by animals, including damage, death and injury caused to people, property and livestock. The owner of a dangerous animal must take precautions to ensure it has no opportunity to inflict damage as stated by this law. If a dog kills or harms farm animals, farmers are entitled to protect the stock in their care. If, for example, a dog is found injuring sheep, the farmer may kill the dog but must report the incident to the police.

Dogs (Fouling of Land) Act 1996

Local authorities and councils use this Act to prevent dogs fouling where there is public access to property or pavements, but allowing exemption of guide dogs for the blind.

Welfare laws

Those keeping animals for commercial reasons:

- Animal Boarding Establishment Act 1963
- Breeding of Dogs Acts 1973, 1991, Breeding and Sale of Dogs (Welfare) Act 1999
- Pet Animals Acts 1951, 1983

Cruelty laws:

- Protection of Animals Acts 1911, 1988
- Protection of Animals (Anaesthetics) Acts 1954, 1982
- Veterinary Surgeons Act 1966

Animal Boarding Establishment Act 1963

The main provision of this Act is that boarding kennels or catteries must be licensed by their local authority in order to trade. The following conditions apply:

- Records must be kept of animal arrivals and departures, and details of owners
- Suitable accommodation must be provided
- Adequate and appropriate supplies of food and water must be available
- Exercise facilities must be provided
- Animals must be protected from disease and risk of fire

In order to ensure that the conditions of the licence are met, the local authority can at any time instruct inspection by an authorised officer or veterinary surgeon. Licences are renewed annually.

Breeding of Dogs Acts 1973, 1991, Breeding and Sale of Dogs (Welfare) Act 1999

The breeding and selling of dogs requires a local authority licence under the 1973 Act, amended by the 1999 Act. In order to gain a licence, animals must be suitably accommodated, fed, exercised and protected from disease and fire. Local authorities have extensive powers to check on the standards of health, welfare and accommodation of these animals. The term 'breeding establishment' refers to any premises where more than two bitches are kept for the purpose of breeding animals for selling. The 1999 Act ensures that 'puppy farms' are regulated by use of recorded information on sales and identification.

In addition, the Breeding of Dogs Act 1991 extended the powers of local authorities to enter any premises and inspect both licensed and unlicensed businesses.

Pet Animals Acts 1951, 1983

This Act was introduced at the end of World War II in response to the worrying number of animals being sold in street markets and pet shops with no restrictions or controls for conditions or care. The Act prohibits the keeping of a pet shop without a licence. A licence is granted after inspection of premises by an approved veterinary surgeon authorised by the local authority. The Act was amended in 1983, making it illegal to sell pets in public places. A licence is granted if the following conditions are met:

- Proper care
- Suitable accommodation
- Housed in the correct conditions with reference to heating, lighting, etc.
- Provided with appropriate food
- Observed and checked at suitable intervals during the day
- Sold only after weaning and a suitable age has been reached
- Prevention of spread of disease
- Emergency and fire precautions for the premises are in place and functional

Protection of Animals Acts 1911–2000

This series of Acts forms the main statutory control on cruelty to a domestic or captive animal. These Acts are used when bringing prosecutions related to animal welfare cases. The Act makes it an offence to cause unnecessary suffering to any domestic or captive animal, either deliberately or by omission (neglect). The Act lists offences such as:

- Inflicting physical cruelty by beating, kicking, etc.
- Inflicting mental cruelty by teasing or terrifying
- Causing unnecessary suffering during transportation by failing to provide food or water at appropriate intervals
- Performing surgery or operations without an anaesthetic
- Poisoning without reason

Protection of Animals (Anaesthetics) Acts 1954, 1982

It is illegal for any operation that will cause pain to be conducted on an animal, unless under anaesthetic (local or general). There are, however, several exceptions to this Act:

- Does not apply to birds, fish or reptiles
- In emergency first-aid situations
- Under permitted Home Office-licensed procedures
- Minor painless operations carried out by a veterinary surgeon or a listed veterinary nurse

Veterinary Surgeons Act 1966

This Act prohibits anyone other than a veterinary surgeon or listed veterinary nurse registered with the Royal College of Veterinary Surgeons from carrying out treatment or operations on animals. The exceptions to this are:

- Minor treatments given by owner, household member or employee of the owner
- Castration or tail docking of lambs, provided they are under a stated age
- Emergency first-aid to maintain life

Animal collection laws

- Welfare of Animals during Transport 1973, 1994 (Amendment) Order 1995
- Abandonment of Animals Act 1960
- Dangerous Wild Animals Act 1976
- Performing Animals (Regulation) Act 1925
- Zoo Licensing Act 1981

Welfare of Animals during Transport 1973, 1994 (Amendment) Order 1995

This order is designed to protect all animals during transport by road, rail, sea and air. Since 1997, a standard set of regulations on journey times, hauliers' journey plans and routes covering EU countries have amended the original order. The regulations cover:

- Loading and unloading of animals
- Housing and containers for transit
- Access to food and water
- Specified number of animals contained together for transit

Abandonment of Animals Act 1960

This Act applies to the abandonment of an animal in circumstances likely to cause it unnecessary suffering. This would apply to an owner or person in control of a companion animal who has abandoned it either completely or for only a temporary period of time.

Dangerous Wild Animals Act 1976, modified 1984 (currently under review)

This Act became necessary when, in the 1960s and 1970s, the public started to keep animals more frequently associated with zoos and safari parks – animals such as leopards, lions, various types of monkey and many other dangerous wild animals. Animals were often kept in poor conditions and insecure housing, causing concern both for their welfare and for people living nearby.

Public demand led to legislation and strict control and inspection by authorised veterinary surgeons who may inspect premises in which these animals are kept. If the inspection is approved, a licence is issued by the local authority.

The Secretary of State has the power to change the list of animals at any time, and any animal on the list is classified as a 'dangerous wild animal'. The Act states that anyone keeping these listed animals must:

- Pay a fee to the local authority for the issue of the licence
- Take out liability insurance
- Provide suitable accommodation
- Be over 18 years of age

Performing Animals (Regulation) Act 1925

A Select Committee of the House of Lords introduced this Act following public concern over the treatment of animals in circuses. As a result, the local authority must be informed of anyone who trains animals for exhibition to the public or exhibits a performing animal to the public, even if it is free of charge, and any such person must be registered to that effect.

The exceptions to this rule are when animals are trained for sporting purposes, military or police work and display.

The Zoo Licensing Act (Amendment) (England & Wales) Regulation 2002 Formerly Zoo Licensing Act 1981

The term 'zoo' refers to the exhibiting of wild animals to the public, for educational purposes. It applies to animal collections that are open to the public for 7 days or more in any year.

This Act was passed after the dramatic increase of zoos and wildlife/safari parks and to include butterfly houses and aquaria. It is intended to protect the zoo animals and the general public by ensuring that standards of care, animal welfare and public safety are in place.

The Act requires licensing by local authorities and inspection by government-listed inspectors.

The welfare of wild animals laws

- The Wildlife and Countryside Acts 1981, 1985
- Convention on International Trade in Endangered Species of Wild Flora and Fauna (CITES) 1973

The Wildlife and Countryside Acts 1981

These Acts replace several existing laws and regulations and cover the protection and conservation of wild animals and their habitats. Land, sea and air-borne species of wild animals are protected. The minister can add to or remove from this list, species which may not legally be injured, killed or taken from the wild.

The Act protects habitats from humans and species in captivity which, if released into the wild, would seriously affect many other species.

The Act brings together and amends existing national legislation and EU directives covering protection of wildlife in the countryside, national parks and other designated areas.

Convention on International Trade in Endangered Species of Wild Flora and Fauna (CITES) 1973

This international agreement helps to protect the world's endangered species by controlling their export and import on a worldwide scale. Animals in this category are:

- Those that are threatened with extinction
- Those likely to become so threatened

Statutory organisations

Royal Society for the Prevention of Cruelty to Animals Act 1932 (RSPCA)

The Society was founded in 1824 by the Reverend Arthur Broome. Its aim is to promote kindness and prevent cruelty to animals. The Act of 1932 empowers the RSPCA to act in certain situations concerning the welfare of animals.

The RSPCA:

- Operates throughout England and Wales, maintaining animal homes and clinics
- Prosecutes in cases of cruelty
- Lobbies on animal welfare issues throughout Europe
- Conducts discreet surveillance of activities, such as livestock transportation abroad

- Funds research into animal welfare
- Maintains links with affiliated organisations in the European community

People's Dispensary for Sick Animals Act 1949 (PDSA)

Founded in 1917 by Maria Dickin, the initial aim of the PDSA was to help sick and injured animals in the east end of London. It provides free veterinary treatment to sick and injured animals when owners are unable to afford treatment. It is not involved with neutering or vaccinations. It has treatment centres and hospitals all over the country, as well as the Pet Aid scheme involving general practices in some counties.

Royal College of Veterinary Surgeons, Veterinary Surgeons Act 1966

The college was established to teach, train and examine people who wished to become registered as veterinary surgeons. In order to remain on the RCVS register, members pay an annual fee. The Act established a council responsible for regulating its membership and ensuring that unqualified people did not use the title of veterinary surgeon, treat or operate on animals.

Veterinary organisations:

- British Small Animal Veterinary Association (BSAVA) exists as an association to promote high standards of medicine and surgery in veterinary practices, continuing education, teaching and research. It provides a forum for discussion of important issues relating to veterinary surgeons, linking back to the RCVS and government departments.
- British Veterinary Association (BVA) is the representative body for the British veterinary profession, providing services and information to members. Members also work for the various divisions of the association, including animal charities (Animal Welfare Foundation), research, education and government service.

Schedule 3 to the Veterinary Surgeons Act has a number of amendments to cover the permitted work of veterinary nurses. The RCVS maintains the statutory list of veterinary nurses and is the awarding body of the veterinary nursing National Vocational Qualifications (NVQs). Qualified veterinary nurses on the list are entitled by law to undertake a range of veterinary treatments and procedures on animals under veterinary direction. The British Veterinary Nursing Association (BVNA) is the national representative body for UK veterinary nurses, liaising closely with the RCVS.

- Unusual body position, e.g. curled up

Chapter 7

Older dogs
- Survive the viraemic stage
- Bloodstained vomit and diarrhoea
- Acute abdominal pain

In some dogs 'blue eye', a clouding of the cornea of the eye, occurs up to three weeks after acute infection.

Vaccination and annual boosters are essential.

Leptospirosis

Also known as Stuttgart disease or Weil's disease in humans, leptospirosis is caused by a filament-like bacterium, *leptospira icterohaemorrhagiae*, which is a zoonone to humans.

The strains that cause the disease in dogs are:

- *Leptospira icterohaemorrhagiae* – (primary host is the rat) attacks mainly the liver
- *Leptospira canicola* – (primary host is the dog) attacks mainly the kidney

These bacteria are easily destroyed by sunlight, disinfectants and temperature extremes.

The disease is spread by direct contact, bite wounds or ingestion of infected food or water. Rodents such as rats are frequently carriers, shedding the bacteria in urine and thus contaminating water.

Incubation is 7–21 days, with severity of the disease caused depending on the susceptibility of the host animal and the strain.

Clinical signs include:

- High temperature
- Shivering and muscle pain
- Vomiting and diarrhoea
- Dehydration
- Shock
- Jaundice (mucous membranes of mouth and eye appear yellow)

Recovered animals shed the bacteria via the urine for some time after recovery. Strict isolation must be observed. Both veterinary surgeon and doctor can provide advice and information to prevent a human carer becoming infected.

An annual booster after initial vaccination is essential.

Rabies

Rabies is caused by a rhabdovirus. It is fragile, surviving for only a short time in the environment, and is destroyed by most disinfectants, heat and light.

Transmitted in the saliva of infected animals, the virus replicates in the muscle cells at the site of infection, then travels via the peripheral nerves to the spinal cord and the brain. Once it is located in the central nervous tissues, neurological signs are observed. The virus also then travels to the salivary glands, where it is shed to infect other mammals, both human and animal. Rabies is therefore a zoonone disease.

Incubation is from 10 days to four months, the time depending on how near to the central nervous system the virus is initially placed. There are three phases or stages to the disease symptoms. However, not all will necessarily occur in all affected animals.

(1) *Preclinical stage* – lasting 2–3 days with a raised body temperature, slow eye reflexes and signs of irritation at the site of the original injury.
(2) *Excitable stage* – lasting up to one week with the animal becoming irritable, aggressive and disorientated, having difficulty standing and epileptic-type fits.
(3) *Dumb stage* – lasting 2–4 days during which the animal becomes progressively paralysed in throat and skeletal muscles, leading to salivation, respiratory difficulties, coma and death.

In some cases the preclinical stage can last for several months during which the virus is shed in the saliva.

Diagnosis is confirmed on postmortem examination of the brain and spinal cord for signs of the virus. Vaccine is available for dogs that live in countries where rabies is endemic or for travelling to a country with rabies in the wild or domestic animal population. The vaccine is given at three months of age and boostered annually.

If bitten by a suspect animal:

• clean the wound immediately using soap or antiseptic solutions
• seek medical attention straight away

Diseases of cats

Infectious feline diseases include:

• Rabies (see Rabies in the dog, p. 116)
• Feline leukaemia
• Feline panleucopenia or feline infectious enteritis
• Chlamydiosis or feline pneumonitis
• Feline viral respiratory disease:
  (a) feline herpesvirus
  (b) feline calicivirus

- Feline infectious anaemia
- Feline infectious peritonitis
- Feline immunodeficiency

Feline leukaemia (FLV)

The retrovirus causing feline leukaemia affects approximately 2% of cats world-wide. It is contagious and, once symptoms appear, almost always fatal. Most cats are exposed to this virus during their life and it is most commonly found where cats are in close contact.

Evidence of the virus is obtained from testing of blood samples using the FLV ELISA test.

The effect of the virus on the host cat depends on the age of the cat when it is infected and the quantity of virus received.

- Some cats become ill and apparently recover
- Some do not become ill and develop an immunity to the disease
- Some develop the disease symptoms after incubation of weeks to several years

Young kittens are most susceptible to the virus. Most die within 2–3 years of exposure or as a result of FLV-related disease conditions, which include:

- Anaemia (lack of red blood cells)
- Lymphosarcoma (tumours of the lymph system)

Clinical signs include:

- High temperature
- Vomiting and diarrhoea
- Weight loss
- Kidney disease
- Enlargement of the spleen

The virus is shed in:

- Saliva
- Faeces
- Urine
- Milk to offspring

The virus is easily destroyed by disinfectants and cannot live long outside a host. Infection can be passed via saliva in bite/fight episodes, contact with other cats or from the mother to the kittens before or after birth via the milk.

The virus replicates in the lymph tissues initially, then moves on to other target systems containing lymph tissue, such as the intestines, causing enteritis, then on to the salivary glands, the urinary and reproductive systems, causing infertility or abortion in pregnant animals.

Control of the disease is via:

- Testing, particularly in multi-cat households
- Animals testing positive being isolated from others
- Disinfection and hygiene in cat areas
- Retesting 12 weeks after positive test to ensure true result
- Testing all new cats that join a household

After two positive tests, the safe choice is to permanently isolate or euthanase the cat. Cats are vaccinated from nine weeks of age with a second dose 2–4 weeks later followed by an annual booster. Before vaccination, all cats are tested for presence of the virus in the blood.

Feline panleucopenia or feline infectious enteritis

Feline panleucopenia is a highly infectious disease of cats, also called:

- Feline parvovirus
- Feline distemper
- Feline infectious enteritis

The disease is caused by a parvovirus, similar to canine parvovirus. The disease can affect cats of any age but is mainly responsible for deaths in young kittens.

The virus is stable and capable of surviving in the environment for months to years and is resistant to most disinfectants. The incubation period is 2–10 days following direct contact with an infected animal or ingestion of the virus. The virus targets rapidly dividing cells and tissues of the small intestines, lymph and bone marrow. It is shed in saliva, vomit, faeces and urine.

Clinical signs include:

- Diarrhoea, often bloodstained
- Dull and listless behaviour
- Abdominal pain
- Fever and dehydration

Blood testing shows a typical reduction in white blood cells (leucopenia), particularly neutrophil white cells.

The virus can cross the placenta during pregnancy and affects the foetus by targeting the brain tissue (cerebellum), causing death or abnormal nervous system development. Kittens show balance difficulties and inco-ordination at about 2–3 weeks of age if affected. If the cat survives the first week of clinical disease, careful nursing can lead to recovery but the intestine may suffer permanent damage, seen as poor absorption of nutrients and constant diarrhoeal episodes.

Vaccination using either live or inactivated vaccine (in pregnant cats) provides good immunity with a booster every 1–2 years.

Chlamydiosis or feline pneumonitis

Chlamydial infection is caused by an organism which lives within cells. Chlamydiae are therefore treated like a virus, but in appearance resemble a bacterium.

Chlamydia cati or *psittaci* affects the conjunctiva of the eye in cats, causing severe conjunctivitis with eye discharges, sneezing and nasal discharge. The conjunctivitis may affect one or both eyes.

Transmission is thought to be via contact with eye/nose discharges, genital tract or gastrointestinal tract secretions from carrier animals. Incubation is 3–10 days.

Clinical signs include:

- Initial watery discharge in one eye, spreading to both
- Inflamed conjunctiva
- Fever
- Rubbing eyes and signs of discomfort
- In kittens, diarrhoea

During pregnancy, chlamydia may cause abortion or stillbirth.

Chlamydiosis may last for 2–3 weeks or longer, especially as a part of the feline viral respiratory disease complex. Recovered animals may shed the responsible organism for several weeks so any treatment usually continues for three weeks postrecovery. The organism is killed by most disinfectants during routine cleaning.

Vaccination is available, boostered annually.

Feline viral respiratory disease

Also known as:

- Cat flu
- Feline upper respiratory disease (FURD)
- Feline viral rhinotracheitis (FVR)

The two main viruses involved are:

- Feline herpesvirus
- Feline calicivirus

Cats are particularly susceptible to infections (both bacterial and viral) of the nose and throat. Due to their location, these infections are called upper respiratory infections or cat flu. While it is essential to vaccinate, as with the 'human flu', vaccines do not protect against some strains of this disease, especially feline calicivirus.

Calicivirus is easily destroyed outside the host by disinfectants. Transmission of the virus is by aerosol or direct contact. As a result of this, any grouping of cats may lead to infection, i.e. shows, boarding, breeding kennels and veterinary surgeries.

Many cats that have survived the disease become carriers, shedding the virus for several years. It is possible to have suspected carrier animals tested by a veterinary surgeon for the presence of the calicivirus.

The incubation period is up to ten days after exposure to high-risk situations (groups of cats) or stress caused by a change to the environment which may lower the cat's resistance to disease.

Clinical signs include:

- Ulcers on the tongue
- Inflammation of the gums
- Unwilling to eat, but producing excess saliva
- High temperature
- Depressed and listless
- Loss of voice

The presence of ulcers may allow bacteria normally present to add to the cat's original symptoms and recovery time.

Feline herpesvirus can survive outside the host for up to eight days. This virus attacks and replicates in the tissues of the respiratory tract and conjunctiva of the eye, causing viral rhinotracheitis. The tissues from nose (*rhino*) to trachea (*tracheitis*) are affected and inflamed, causing breathing difficulties, sneezing and coughing. Recovered animals can act as carriers, shedding the virus particularly when stressed.

Viral rhinotracheitis is the most serious form of upper respiratory disease, often leaving recovered animals with damage to the nasal passages. This causes the affected cat to periodically sneeze, snuffle and have a runny nose, the discharge occasionally being thick with pus.

The incubation period is from two to ten days postexposure.

Clinical signs include:

- High temperature
- Discharge from eyes and nose, later becoming thickened due to bacterial infection
- Depressed and listless
- Loss of appetite

- Sneezing
- Conjunctivitis
- Mouth ulcers
- Pneumonia
- Abortion in pregnant queens

Vaccine is available, boostered annually by intranasal methods. In high-risk situations, six-monthly administration is advisable.

Feline infectious anaemia

Infectious anaemia is the direct loss of red blood cells caused by a blood parasite called *Haemobartonella felis or Eperythrozoon felis*. Transmission is thought to be by bloodsucking parasites, e.g. the flea. Cats of all ages can be affected. When the disease is linked to feline leukaemia, affecting white blood cell numbers, the recovery is poor.

The single-celled parasite responsible can be demonstrated on a blood smear examination in the laboratory. Discussion with a veterinary surgeon is essential at this time. Products to safely remove fleas from the affected household are required and other cats in the same household may need to be examined and treated.

Incubation is up to 50 days, with recovered or carrier animals often shedding the parasite for months.

Clinical signs include:

- Pale mucous membranes – mouth and gums
- Breathing difficulty
- Listless and loss of appetite
- Third eyelid up as a sign of ill health
- High temperature
- Weight loss

Animals respond well to treatment using specific antibiotics. There is no vaccine against this virus.

Feline infectious peritonitis

Also called feline infectious vasculitis, infectious peritonitis is caused by a coronavirus which affects mostly young cats under three years of age. It causes the lining membrane of the abdomen (peritoneum) and contents to become inflamed (peritonitis). This disease is not limited in effect to the organs of the abdomen and may also affect the nervous system and eyes.

Contact between cats via urine and faeces carrying the shed virus will act as the transmission method. Carrier animals may carry the virus for years, with mothers possibly passing the disease to their kittens. The virus is unstable outside the body and easily destroyed by disinfectants.

Diseased cats are sometimes affected by feline leukaemia, which may make them susceptible to the peritonitis virus. The form taken by the disease will vary depending on the ability of the individual's immune system to mount a response to the virus challenge.

Clinical signs include:

- Lack of appetite and gradual weight loss
- Fever
- Swollen abdomen due to fluid accumulation
- Diarrhoea and vomiting

Later signs include:

- Organ failure
- Neurological signs including inability to stand, paralysis and convulsions
- Inflammation within the structure of the eye, affecting sight

Depending on the form taken by the disease, it is often further described as *wet* (fluid in body cavities) or *dry* (tumour-like masses called granulomatous lesions forming on organs).

Control of the disease is by strict hygiene and disinfection particularly in multi-cat households or where groups of cats are housed. There is no vaccine available in the UK at present.

Feline immunodeficiency

Feline immunodeficiency is caused by a virus of the lentivirus group. The disease is often characterised by a long incubation period. Incubation to signs of the disease can initially take four weeks and finally several years; as a result, it is unusual to find the infection in cats under two years of age. The disease attacks the lymph system, causing a suppression of the body's immune response. Initially the disease was known as T-lymphotrophic T cell lentivirus, due to the effect on the cells of the immune system (T cells and B cells).

The virus is carried in the saliva of the infected animal and transmitted by bite. Therefore cats that have access to outdoor life are more at risk than those housed completely indoors. Male cats are more commonly infected due to territorial fighting.

Commercial screening kits are available to detect antibodies to the virus from a blood sample. After the initial body response to the virus, the cat shows signs of the disease within a few weeks. These signs are very similar to those of feline leukaemia and include:

- Conjunctivitis and nasal discharge
- Enlarged superficial lymph nodes (*lymphadenopathy*)
- Mouth and gum inflammation
- Diarrhoea
- Skin problems
- High temperature
- Neurological signs that include difficulty in walking and change in temperament

The animal then appears to recover but due to gradual suppression of its immune responses, it will frequently suffer from recurring or ongoing infections of various kinds, often failing to respond to veterinary treatment. The cat will suffer weight loss, becoming inactive and listless.

There is no vaccine available so owners are advised to castrate male cats and limit exposure to other neighbourhood cats in order to avoid contact with an infected animal.

Immunity

Immunity refers to the body's natural protection against life-threatening disease. It can be achieved by:

- Contracting the disease and recovering
- Vaccination

The purpose of a vaccination programme is to prevent the disease by preventing or limiting the infection in a host animal. Vaccines cause stimulation of the immune system which in turn produces *antibodies*. The cells of the immune system responsible for producing this protection are the B-lymphocytes and these in turn are assisted by the T-lymphocytes. Both are white blood cells, which may be targeted and destroyed by certain viruses. The antibodies will recognise specific viruses or bacteria and prevent or limit their ability to produce disease in the host animal.

At the time of vaccination, the veterinary surgeon will fully examine the animal to ensure that adverse conditions which may influence the manner in which the body responds to the vaccine are not present, such as a high body temperature indicating infection.

There are many factors which influence an animal's ability to respond to vaccination. These include:

- Presence of colostral antibodies from the mother's milk which could interfere with the vaccine
- Vaccine type

- Route of administration – subcutaneous or intranasal
- Animal's age
- Medication that could interfere with the vaccine, i.e. anti-inflammatory drugs
- Diet
- Infection already present

Immunity may be acquired by passive or active means. Passive immunity results from the transfer of maternal antibodies to the newborn via the colostrum in the milk. The degree of immunity depends on the quantity of the first milk let down and the quality of the mother's own antibodies resulting from her recent vaccinations. Passive immunity lasts only as long as the antibodies remain active in the blood, from three to 12 weeks. After this time the body will eliminate the antibodies.

Active immunity develops either as a result of the animal becoming infected with a micro-organism, developing the disease and recovering or from a vaccination. Both cause the body to react in much the same manner by stimulating the production of antibodies which are specific to particular microbes (*pathogens* or *antigens*).

Vaccines are prepared from live or inactivated (killed) preparations of micro-organisms. They stimulate the immune system of the vaccinated animal to produce antibodies to specific disease-producing materials.

Chapter 11
Zoonones

Also known as zoonoses, these diseases are transmissible from animals to people. Most domestic animals can transmit zoonones.

Dogs

Dog infection	Disease in humans
Leptospirosis	Weil's disease
Toxocariasis	Visceral larval migrans
Echinococcosis	Hydatid disease
Sarcoptic mange	Skin rash and bites
Cheyletiella mites	Skin rash and bites
Ringworm	Skin lesions and hair loss
Salmonellosis	Diarrhoea/vomiting
Rabies	Rabies (hydrophobia)

Cats

Human disease	Signs
Pasteurellosis	Bites or scratches become infected
Cat scratch fever	High temperature, flu-like signs, rash
Ringworm (Fig. 11.1)	Raised, circular, inflamed skin lesion
Toxoplasmosis	Abortion of foetus
Rabies	Fever, itching at original bite area, behaviour changes, paralysis and death

Zoonones from other species

Disease	Microbe	Species
Brucellosis	Bacteria	Cattle
Campylobacter	Bacteria	Hamsters

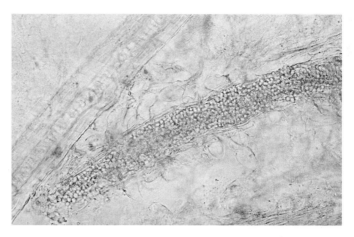

Fig. 11.1 Ringworm spores on a hair shaft.

Psittacosis	Bacteria	Birds
Salmonellosis	Bacteria	Mice, rats and guinea pigs
Tetanus	Bacteria	Horses and other herbivores

Prevention of zoonones

In order to minimise the risk to people of diseases which can be passed by companion animals, the following simple but effective hygiene precautions must be taken:

- Investigate any signs of illness.
- Control fleas and worms.
- Vaccinate animals.
- Do not allow pets to lick children's faces.
- Wash hands after handling any animal.
- Do not feed pets from household plates or dishes.
- Use separate utensils for food preparation.
- Daily collection and safe disposal of faeces.
- Always wear gloves when handling body discharges.

Chapter 12
Parasitology

A *parasite* lives in or on another living body. The parasite benefits by taking nourishment from the host, which can be any species.

Parasitology terms

- *Transport host* – transports the parasite to the next host. No development takes place in the parasite
- *Paratenic host* – same as transport but the parasite must be eaten, in order to be excreted and passed on to the next host
- *Intermediate host* – some parasites must spend time on/in this host in order to develop to their next life cycle stage
- *Final host* – host in which the parasite completes its development
- *Permanent parasite* –develops through all life stages and lives on one host
- *Temporary parasites* – move from host to host
- *Endoparasite* – lives inside the host's body
- *Ectoparasite* – lives on the surface of the host's body

The parasite feeds on the host but does not deliberately kill it, as this would destroy its food source. Some hosts may die as a result of the parasite's feeding activities or from toxins released by it.

In order to prevent disease or death of the host species, control of parasites is important. Routine control in equine and large animals is necessary to keep parasite numbers down. Control in small animals (dogs, cats, rabbits, etc.) aims to completely remove all parasites, whether internal or external. There are many easy-to-use and effective products for removing external parasites such as fleas and lice, with a residue effect which will last for varying periods of time. The products supplied for eliminating internal parasites are collectively called *anthelmintics*.

External parasites

Flea – Ctenocephalides (Fig. 12.1)

- Adult fleas can live for two years without feeding
- Flea eggs hatch in 1–2 days

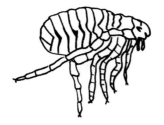

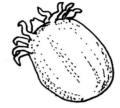

Fig. 12.2 Tick – *Ixodes*.

Fig. 12.1 Flea – *Ctenocephalides*.

- Flea larvae feed for 4–8 days (in carpets or bedding)
- Larvae spin cocoons and adults emerge in five days or less
- Adult flea cycle may take only three weeks, but if the environment is unsuitable, the larval stage can last for months

Tick – Ixodes (Fig. 12.2)

- Adult tick can live for two years without feeding
- Engorged female can lay 1000–3000 eggs
- Larva hatches in 30 days
- Nymphs emerge from moulted larva
- Adult tick emerges after 12 days
- Feeding is required between each stage of development

Diseases are transmitted in the saliva of the tick to other host animals. These diseases include:

- **Lyme disease** – a bacterial tick-borne infection caused by *Borrelia burgdorferi*. The bacteria can cause skin discolouration, cardiac and joint disease in the infected animal. It is endemic in a number of states in the USA. It is also carried in Europe by ticks of wildlife hosts, such as rodents and deer. Signs:
  - sudden onset of lameness with arthritic pain in one or more joints (i.e. carpal or wrist joint) which may last only a few days, recurring at intervals
  - high temperature with enlarged surface lymph nodes

- **Ehrlichiosis** – caused by a parasite which lives inside certain white blood cells. It is transmitted by ticks during feeding on the host animal's blood. It is found in the Mediterranean basin in Europe and other Mediterranean countries. The severity and recovery of the host animal depends on the activity of its immune system. Certain breeds of dog are particularly susceptible to the disease, e.g. German shepherds. Babesiosis may also be present, having been passed by the tick at the same time. Signs:
  - high temperature and inappetance

- lymph nodes enlarged
- bleeding from the nose and under the skin
- anaemia

- **Babesiosis** – caused by a protozoan that develops and multiplies in the tick salivary glands, from which it is transmitted to the host animal during feeding. It is endemic across much of Europe. The parasitic protozoa infect red blood cells. The severity of the disease varies, depending on the species and strain of *Babesia* and the health status of the infected animal. Signs:
  - pale mucous membranes
  - anaemia
  - breathing problems and collapse

Mite – Sarcoptes

Causes sarcoptic mange.

- Sarcoptic mite may live only 3–4 weeks
- Eggs are laid by the burrowing female (burrows into the epidermal skin layer)
- Larvae hatch in 3–5 days
- Nymph follows, through two nymph stages
- Adult mite emerges. The full cycle takes about 17 days

Lice

	Dog	**Cat**
Biting louse	*Trichodectes*	*Felicola substratus*
Sucking louse	*Linognathus*	

- Eggs are laid and cemented to the coat hair of the host. Eggs are called *nits*
- Three stages of nymph emerge
- Adult emerges after last nymph moult, after three weeks

Fur mite – Cheyletiella

- Often referred to as 'walking dandruff'. There are many different types, living on the skin cells and tissue fluid of the host to gain nutrients
- Eggs are laid and cemented to coat hair, similar to lice
- Eggs hatch into six-legged larvae
- Moult into eight-legged larvae
- Adult stage is reached

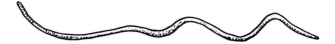

Fig. 12.3 Roundworm.

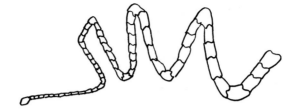

Fig. 12.4 Tapeworm.

Internal parasites

Endoparasites for small animals are divided into two groups:

(1) Roundworms (nematodes) (Fig. 12.3):
    (a)   are unsegmented
    (b)   have a body cavity
    (c)   have an alimentary tract throughout
(2) Tapeworms (cestodes) (Fig. 12.4):
    (a)   are segmented
    (b)   each segment is independent
    (c)   have a complete alimentary tract in each segment

Infected animals do not always show signs of infestation, which only start to appear if the infestation becomes overwhelming to the health of the host animal:

- Scooting on bottom (anal irritation)
- Constantly hungry and eating (*polyphagia*)
- Weight loss
- Vomiting and diarrhoea seen in heavy infestation
- Unhealthy, dull coat
- Enlarged abdomen

Common worms in the UK include:

- Roundworms
    (a)   *Toxocara canis*
    (b)   *Toxocara cati*

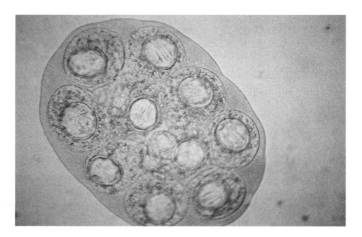

Fig. 12.5 *Dipylidium caninum* worm egg.

- Tapeworms
  (a) *Dipylidium caninum*
  (b) *Echinococcus granulosus*

Life cycles

Tapeworm – Dipylidium caninum

This tapeworm affects both dogs and cats and has an intermediate host, which is the flea.

(1) Animal passes egg-filled tapeworm segments in its faeces (Fig. 12.5)
(2) The segments burst, releasing individual eggs that are eaten by the flea larvae
(3) During grooming the animal swallows the tapeworm-carrying flea larvae
(4) The tapeworm matures in the animal host
(5) The adult tapeworm releases mature, egg-filled segments and, if the host is not treated with anthelmintic drugs, the cycle begins again

Roundworm – Toxocara canis

This worm is a zoonone. It can migrate in human tissues and is linked to a disease called toxocariasis in humans, which can cause blindness in children.

(1) Infective eggs or larval forms of this roundworm are swallowed by the dog
(2) They migrate to the body tissues, often migrating to developing fetuses
(3) They localise in the intestines, moving to the unborn before the end of pregnancy or infecting them through the mother's milk after birth

(4)   The larvae now mature, passing eggs in the puppies' faeces

(5)   These are swallowed by other puppies or the mother, and the cycle repeats unless the dogs are treated

Prevention of toxocariasis

- Worm animals regularly
- Control the intermediate hosts (fleas and lice)
- Dispose of faeces immediately
- Disinfect where faeces have been
- Always wash hands thoroughly
- Wash animals' bowls separately from human utensils
- Do not let the animal lick your face
- Keep the animal's anal area clean
- Examine faeces regularly for signs of worms

Chapter 13
Hygiene

Disinfectants and antiseptics

These chemicals play an important role in maintaining the health and/or promoting the recovery of an animal. Their use in basic hygiene for housing, kennels, catteries or in veterinary practice hospitals is important to the care of both the environment and living tissues. These products are chemicals which, if used incorrectly, such as at low concentrations, allow micro-organisms to develop a resistance, thus reducing their value.

Some of these chemicals are designed for use on the environment and non-living structures, others are designed for use on living tissue.

Hygiene terms

- *Sterilisation* – the removal or destruction of all living micro-organisms including bacterial spores.
- *Asepsis* – is a state of being free from micro-organisms.
- *Disinfectants* – are referred to as *bactericidal*, i.e. they will kill micro-organisms.
- *Antiseptics* – are referred to as *bacteriostatic*, i.e. they will prevent organisms from multiplying and therefore infections cannot develop.

Principles of disinfection

Disinfectants are used on the environment only, on surfaces like floors, housing walls and ceilings and runs. Disinfectants are harmful to living tissues so if they are used in the workplace or at home, protective clothing (gloves and in some cases masks) should be worn.

Antiseptics are used to disinfect hands prior to operating, before handling animals to prevent transfer of microbes and after handling contaminated material. They are also used to disinfect the patient's skin before and after surgery or after injury.

Disinfectants

Properties of an ideal disinfectant:

- Effective against a wide range of micro-organisms
- Non-toxic to animals or humans
- Non-staining to animals' coats or housing
- Has a good wetting ability and penetrates organic material attached to surfaces
- Stable in storage and has a good shelf-life
- Only low concentrations are necessary for effect
- Economical and readily available

Disinfectants are most effective when:

- Used with hot water rather than cold
- Left in contact with surfaces for the correct amount of time (see instructions on label)
- Used at correct strength
- Not mixed with other chemicals
- Freshly prepared (see instructions on label)

Disinfectants can be inactivated by:

- Organic materials from the body, e.g. blood, faeces, pus and urine
- Surfaces, e.g. cork, wood and plastic
- Materials, e.g. wool or cotton
- Excess minerals in water (hard water areas)
- Mixing disinfectants and detergent

When choosing a disinfectant for the cleaning of housing and surfaces, care is needed. Some products are toxic to certain species of animals. The phenols or phenol-containing compounds are toxic to cats, rabbits and rodents so they tend to be used only in large animal and farming industry facilities. Products in this group are recognised as black, white or clear. They normally have a strong and distinctive smell and will stain housing and bedding materials. Examples are Jeyes Fluid, Izal, Stericol, Ibcol, Phisohex and Dettol.

Disinfectants for environmental use only destroy the micro-organism by disrupting its cell wall or contents in such a way that the microbe will die or be killed by the chemical. The most resistant microbes are:

- Bacterial spores
- Some viruses (unenveloped)

The least resistant microbes are:

- Some viruses (enveloped)
- Bacteria (vegetative)
- Fungi

The most effective disinfectants include:

- Aldehydes
- Peroxides
- Halogens (iodines and chlorines)

Aldehydes (formaldehyde and glutaraldehyde) (e.g. Formula H, Parvocide and Vetcide)

These are effective against a wide range of micro-organisms but hazardous to living tissue. Never use on living tissues in any form.

Care must be taken while mixing, using and discarding solutions. Avoid contact with skin or eyes and inhaling the fumes. Use these compounds only if necessary and follow work-based safety guidelines for safe use.

Powdered peroxygen or oxidising agents (peroxides) (e.g. Vircon)

These are effective against a wide range of micro-organisms. They are available in a powder form, which is mixed with water as directed by the manufacturer. The solution is used for disinfection of surfaces and housing. It is considered safe in contact with skin but protective clothes and gloves should be worn, as with all other chemicals. Once mixed, it is stable as a disinfectant for five days. Discard old solution and make up fresh as instructed.

Halogen group (chlorine release compounds) (e.g. hyperchlorites like household bleach and products like Halamid)

An effective disinfectant if correctly used. Always follow dilution instructions for best effect as this chemical can be inactivated by incorrect dilution and by organic materials.

It is very irritant to tissues so extreme care should be taken in preparation, use and disposal. Thoroughly rinse off any surface that has been in contact with this disinfectant. The product loses activity on exposure to air and light. New dilutions should be made up frequently.

Iodophors – see antiseptics (Pevidine)

Iodine

This is used on surfaces as a solution of water or alcohol. It is effective against a wide range of micro-organisms but can be inactivated by organic matter. It will also stain surfaces and materials.

Antiseptics (used as skin cleaners)

When applied to skin or mucous membranes of living tissues, antiseptics stop or prevent the growth of micro-organisms like bacteria and fungi but will not necessarily kill microbes.

Quaternary ammonium compounds (QACs) (a) chlorhexidine plus a detergent property, e.g. Hibiscrub or Dinex; (b) cetrimide, e.g. Cetavlon, Savlon or Vetasep

These are effective against microbes and have a rapid action as an antiseptic. They are often used as a preoperative skin cleaner and as a surgeon's scrub. They have a low toxicity to tissues but may be irritant to some individuals. Recontamination by microbes is prevented for a time due to a residual effect. Use at recommended dilution and only on intact skin.

Iodophors – iodine-based compounds (e.g. Pevidine scrub, Betadine)

These are effective against skin microbes, non-irritant and have low toxicity to tissues. Their action is slow so length of time in contact with the skin surface is important. Follow instructions for use.

Disinfecting housing or surfaces

To maximise the effect of the chemicals being used and to prevent inactivation by organic materials, the following rules apply:

(1)   Remove animal, food bowls, toys and bedding.
(2)   Soak all surfaces with hot, soapy water.
(3)   Scrub the soaked surfaces with bristle brush.
(4)   Wash and rinse away all materials and soap.
(5)   Apply the disinfectant at correct dilution and for correct time.
(6)   Rinse all trace of disinfectant off with water and hose down.
(7)   Leave to dry.

Chapter 14
Basic Nutrition

Food or nutrients are required by the body in order to produce energy. Energy is necessary to drive the essential processes and systems in the body.

- Breathing
- Circulating the blood to tissues and cells
- Maintaining body temperature
- Muscle movement throughout the body
- The materials for repair, growth and reproduction
- General health

Nutrients are any food products that will support life. There are six major groups:

- Those that can supply energy:
  (1) protein
  (2) carbohydrates
  (3) fats
- Those which do not supply energy but are needed for its production:
  (4) vitamins
  (5) minerals
  (6) water

Animals eat in order to satisfy their energy needs. In the wild, when animals have eaten enough food to meet the body's energy demands, they will stop. However, due to the improved taste of pet foods, scraps from the human table and 'treats', some companion animals will eat in excess of their body's needs, resulting in obesity and other linked diseases. Many animals have a sedentary lifestyle with owners unable to provide sufficient exercise, which means that nutrients in excess of body needs will be converted to storage as body fat (*adipose tissue*).

Protein

(a) Animal origin
  - meat
  - fish
  - eggs
  - milk

(b) Vegetable origin
  - soya and other pulses/beans
  - cereals

Proteins are large molecules, consisting of hundreds of single units called *amino acids* which join together as chains. Dietary protein is broken down during the digestive process into amino acids. Proteins are made up of a combination of 23 amino acids. Animals need all 23 amino acids in order to maintain their body proteins. Some are obtained from food and some are made within the body.

Dogs require ten amino acids to be supplied by the diet and can create or synthesise the remainder. Cats require 11 amino acids to be supplied via the diet. The extra one (compared to dogs) cannot be synthesised by the cat and can only be obtained from animal protein. These dietary amino acids are referred to as *essential*.

Amino acids

- Arginine
- Histidine
- Isoleucine
- Leucine
- Lysine
- Methionine
- Phenylalanine
- Taurine (which the cat is unable to synthesise)
- Threonine
- Tryptophan
- Valine

Function

- Energy (only used as an energy source if in excess or other energy sources are not available)
- Growth
- Repair of tissues

- Immune system to protect from disease
- Assisting metabolic reactions (enzyme and hormone)

Deficiency

- Poor growth
- Weight loss
- Disease

Many tissues in the body rely on protein as a major component, e.g. hormones, enzymes, plasma proteins and antibodies. The quantities required by each animal will vary depending on:

- Species
- Age
- Sex
- Quality of the protein

The higher the biological value of a protein (in other words, the easier it is for the body to use), the smaller the quantity required. High-value protein includes:

- Egg
- White meat (chicken)
- Fish

Low-value protein includes:

- Soya bean and other pulses
- Cereals

Excess protein in the diet cannot be stored but is converted by the liver to energy and nitrogenous waste (urea). This is then removed from the body by the kidneys.

Carbohydrate

(a) Animal origin
  - milk
(b) Vegetable origin
  - cereal starches (oats, lentils, rice)
  - root vegetables (potatoes)

Carbohydrate can be divided into digestible (starches) and indigestible (dietary fibre or cellulose). Dietary fibre is found in plants and cereals and provides bulk to the faecal materials. It assists in regulating bowel function and the movement of undigested nutrients through the digestive tract.

Function

- Energy
- Provides dietary fibre

Deficiency

- None, provided other energy nutrients are available in the diet (i.e. fats or proteins)

Carbohydrate is broken down in the digestive tract to simple sugars which are essential for most of the body's energy. If simple sugars are unavailable as a nutrient, the body can divert some amino acids to become an energy source.

If the diet contains more carbohydrate than required for the production of energy, the surplus is converted into body fat and stored as adipose tissue.

Simple sugars can be converted into a temporary stored form called *glycogen*. This is stored in the liver and muscles and converted back to simple sugar whenever its energy is needed by the body.

Fats

(a) Animal origin
- milk and other dairy produce
- fish oil
- fat of body origin (attached to meat)

(b) Vegetable origin
- nuts
- seed oils, i.e. sunflower, oil seed rape, linseed
- margarine

Function

- Energy (a very concentrated form)
- Improved taste to the diet
- For the absorption, transport and storage of the fat-soluble vitamins – A, D, E and K
- Provide essential fatty acids for body use

Table 14.1 Fat-soluble vitamins.

Vitamin	Source	Function
A (retinol)	Fish oils, liver, egg and cereals	Night vision, body cell division
D (cholecalciferol)	Liver, fish oils, egg and cereals	Regulates calcium levels, bone growth and repair
E (tocopherol)	Vegetable oils, egg and cereals	Supports tissues and cells around the body
K	Developed in the intestines (no need for dietary source), green vegetables	Assists in blood clotting

Deficiency

- Reproduction problems
- Impaired wound healing
- Poor coat condition
- Dry skin

Fat is also called *lipid*. It is made up of glycerol, with attached fatty acids. Fatty acids are a very concentrated form of energy compared to protein or carbohydrates.

In the dog and cat there are three essential fatty acids: linoleic, arachidonic and linolenic. Provided there is a dietary source, the dog can obtain or synthesise all three from any type of dietary fat. The cat, however, is only able to synthesise one essential fatty acid from the diet and must therefore be provided with a dietary source of the other two. Combined with the need to be supplied with one of the amino acids in the dietary food, this means the cat is considered a true carnivore. That is, it cannot maintain full health without a diet of animal tissues to utilise as a source of ready-made essential fatty or amino acids.

Body fat (adipose tissue) is created from a combination of fatty acids and simple sugars, if either is in excess in the diet.

Vitamins

Vitamins are important in the chemical reactions that go to make up metabolism. There are two groups:

- Fat-soluble vitamins – A, D, E and K (Table 14.1)
- Water-soluble vitamins – B complex group and vitamin C (Table 14.2)

Fat-soluble vitamins are stored in fatty tissues and in the liver; and therefore could reach dangerous levels if given in excess. Water-soluble vitamins are not

Table 14.2   Water-soluble vitamins.

Vitamin	Source	Function
B$_1$ (thiamine)	Cereals, organ meat, green vegetables, dairy products	Assists metabolic reactions, i.e. converts sugars to fatty tissues
B$_2$ (riboflavin)	Organ meats, milk	Use and release of energy by cells
B$_6$ (pyridoxine)	Cereals, meat and yeast	Metabolism of amino acids
B$_{12}$ (cyanocobalamin)	Fish, organ meats	Blood cell production in bone marrow
Folic acid	Organ meats, fish; synthesised by gut	Blood cell production in bone marrow
Biotin	Produced by gut bacteria	Assists body metabolism
C, ascorbic acid	Green vegetables; created in the body	Creates collagen for tissues, supports bone cells

Dogs and cats may synthesise most vitamin C required by the body, but primates, fish and guinea-pigs are unable to do so and must receive a dietary source for body health and function.

stored and must be supplied continuously via the diet, and supplemented in medical conditions that lead to water loss, i.e. diarrhoea. Most species can produce vitamin C in the liver, but the guinea-pig cannot and must be given vitamin C supplements routinely.

Minerals

```
(a)  Animal origin
     •  dairy products
     •  meat
     •  egg
     •  bone meal
(b)  Vegetable origin
     •  cereals
     •  green vegetables
     •  salt
```

These are important for a variety of functions in the body. They are often referred to as *ash* on containers of pet food.

Provided the animal is fed a balanced dietary product, minerals do not normally need to be supplemented.

Minerals are divided into two groups:

(1) Macro- or major minerals (needed in large or regular amounts):
- calcium
- chloride
- magnesium
- phosphorus
- potassium
- sodium

(2) Trace minerals (needed in only small amounts):
- copper
- iodine
- iron
- selenium
- zinc

Function

- Assist maintenance of pH balance in the body
- Maintain the body's fluid balance
- Essential for the function of muscle tissues and conducting nerve impulses
- Help regulate the body's metabolism (via enzymes and hormones)

Never feed any one product in excess within an otherwise balanced diet. Deficiencies in minerals are often associated with excess minerals being added to the diet, i.e. calcium deficiencies can be caused by phosphorus excess in the diet. This could happen in animals being fed an excess of dietary meat or organ tissues.

Table 14.3 Minerals.

Mineral	Food Source	Function
Calcium	Milk, cheese, meat and bone	Nerve cell repair, muscle and bone formation
Sodium	Salt and cereals	Nerve and muscle activity, fluid balance in the body
Magnesium	Bone, cereals and greens	Bone formation and synthesis of protein
Phosphorus	Milk, meat and bones	Bone and teeth formation
Copper	Bones and meat	Red blood cell formation – haemoglobin
Iodine	Milk and fish	Formation of hormone from thyroid gland
Iron	Meat, eggs and greens	Red blood cell formation – haemoglobin
Selenium	Fishmeal, meat and cereals	Synthesis of vitamin E
Zinc	Meat and cereals	Tissue maintenance and aids digestion of food

If a good-quality diet (either commercial product or home recipe) is being fed, there should be no need to supplement vitamins and minerals to an normal healthy animal.

Water

Water is essential for all cells in the body and is found inside and outside all cells; 60–70% of body weight is water. It is involved with nearly every body process. As a result of the presence of water in the body, the following can take place:

- Transport of any material between tissues/cells
- Electrolyte balance
- pH balance
- Control of temperature
- Lubrication of all tissue cells
- A medium for blood and lymph

Water cannot be stored by the body and must be available all the time for all animals. Water in the body comes from:

- Food
- Drinking
- Chemical reactions (metabolism)

Water is lost:

- In urine
- Via the lungs in breathing
- In faeces
- In sweat via the skin

It is important to stress that *fresh water must be available at all times*. This must be emphasised to all pet owners. Some water will be available from canned food, but if a dry diet is given, the animal must receive water by drinking.

General considerations for feeding

- There are major differences in the dietary needs of each species of animal
- If the diet is balanced for that species, do not supplement vitamins or minerals
- The diet should provide enough energy for the animal, supplied by fats and carbohydrate rather than by diverting protein

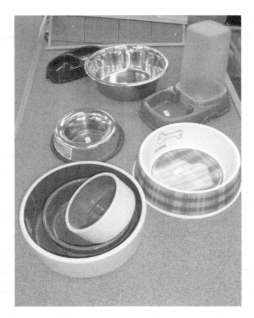

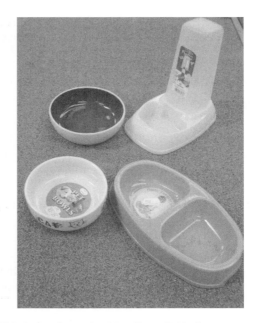

Fig. 14.1 Some food bowls available for dogs.   **Fig. 14.2** Some food bowls available for cats.

- Energy levels and requirements will vary with age or life stages and activity levels
- Read instructions carefully before feeding dry diets in particular. Use a recommended 'measure' for quantities to prevent overfeeding

Figures 14.1 and 14.2 show a variety of food bowls available for the pet dog and cat.

Life stages for nutrition of the dog and cat

The main dietary components are:

- protein
- carbohydrate
- essential fats
- vitamins and minerals

These components provide energy following their breakdown in the gut and absorption. However, fat will provide twice as much energy as protein and carbohydrates. The quantities of the main components can be adjusted for any life stage in order to meet the demand of the animal (i.e. during growth phase, pregnancy and lactation) provided that the basic rules are understood.

Food provides energy but it is important that the nutrient content is balanced to the individual animal's requirements. The following stages need to be considered for the dog and cat:

- Growing puppies and kittens
- Adult maintenance
- Working dogs
- Senior dog and cat
- Pregnancy

Nutritional differences between the dog and the cat

Dog

Dogs are not true carnivores (meat eating); they have retained a number of molar teeth for chewing and grinding food which demonstrate this. Dogs can convert vegetable protein and fat into the ingredients necessary for body function. However, a vegetarian diet may not be balanced enough to maintain health in the long term. How the food supplied tastes, its energy content and its digestibility all need to be considered. A complete diet allows the animal to maintain body weight and fitness by supply of all the essential nutrients to meet whatever the daily needs of the animal may be.

Commercial proprietary diet types:

- *Canned food* – meat and vegetable protein-based foods to be mixed with dog biscuits or meal for a complete diet
- *Complete semi-moist food* – similar to canned but can contain three times the calories of canned foods
- *Complete dry food* – have nearly all the water content removed, leaving them more concentrated than semi-moist foods, and containing four times the calorie content of canned food. Some may need re-hydrating with water before being fed to the dog
- *Biscuits* – these are cereal-based (providing carbohydrates) but also contain high levels of fat, vitamins, minerals and small quantities of protein
- *Treats* – are used for reward or snacks, and are often very high in calories, colour and smell

Cat

The cat is unusual, having remained completely carnivorous (known as an obligate carnivore), as a result protein will supply the majority of its energy requirements. This means that the dietary protein requirements for a cat are considerably higher than for a dog.

Commercial proprietary diet types:

- *Canned/foil-contained foods* – are meat or fish based, with some cereal (carbohydrates), fat, vitamins, and minerals for a complete diet. The protein levels are much higher than in dog food.
- *Soft moist foods* – are supplied in pellet form containing meat, soya protein, and some fats. These are usually packed in foil sachets.
- *Dry food* – resembles small biscuits containing fish and meat as a base, cereals, vitamins and minerals, but tend to be low in fats. Fresh water must always be available for a cat fed on this form of diet.

All commercial proprietary diets and biscuit meal have full instructions for feeding, outlining quantities for all breeds and sizes.

Home-made diets

Home-made recipes for dogs and cats must still form a balanced diet. These can be time consuming to prepare. It is important to either mince or chop up food into small pieces for a cat diet because cats are unable to chew, they can only hold and tear food.

Examples of food source in a home-made diet for a dog would include:

- Proteins
  - liver (high in phosphorus but low in calcium, rich in vitamins A and B)
  - heart (high in fat, therefore used only in small quantities)
  - chicken and turkey are lower in calories than other meats and easily digested
  - fish is a good protein source but all bones must be removed (grill or steam but do not boil)
  - egg (scrambled) is useful for recovery from illness and restoring appetite
  - minced beef or lamb will include animal fat
- Vegetables (seasoned, cooked carrot, cabbage and green beans) provide fibre, vitamins and minerals
- Pasta, noodles and potato are good sources of carbohydrate but need flavouring

---

Feeding guidelines

(1) Never feed bones of any kind
(2) Feed a good-quality food product
(3) Remove uneaten food daily
(4) Always provide fresh water, changed daily
(5) Check that the protein levels are correct for the animal's life stage and circumstance (to prevent upset to the gut and diarrhoea)
(6) Serve food at room temperature for a dog and slightly warmed for a cat
(7) Never feed raw egg white (a chemical in it makes biotin unavailable)

Table 14.4 Sources of nutrients.

Nutrient	Source
Protein	Muscle meat, milk, eggs, pulses
Fat	Animal fat, vegetable oils, some meats
Carbohydrate	Cereal, potato, pasta, rice

Nutritional balance

All foods supply energy. This is measured in units of heat (kJ/g or kcal/g). The foods of a dog or cat diet which provide protein, fat and carbohydrate (Table 14.4) all contribute energy. Protein and carbohydrate are equal in energy content, but fat will provide twice this amount of energy gram for gram weight.

The protein content of a diet must make up at least 20% of the total energy present in the diet in order for enough to be eaten for body maintenance needs.

Dogs and cats make use of fat in their diet. It is a rich source of energy and is required for the essential fatty acids (EFA) needed for functions in the body. Fat is also stored as tissue around the body if fed in excess, to be used when food becomes short.

Carbohydrate is not required by the dog or cat but is used as a source of energy from cooked starches and sugars released from cereals, potatoes or pasta.

Supplementation

Supplementation refers to foods that are provided as well as the normal ration and diet (Figs 14.3 and 14.4). While some supplements may correct a deficiency in an animal with a medical disease, others may be used as:

- Treats
- To increase food intake
- As a reward during training

Supplementation should not be used to improve a poor diet or be supplied in excess. A good-quality complete and balanced food will provide the nutrients required for health and fitness.

Growing puppies and kittens

After weaning, puppies and kittens need to be supplied, in their daily diet, with about 2–2½ times the nutrients required by an adult of the same breed/species.

These increased requirements will gradually decrease as the animal becomes older and reaches adult weight.

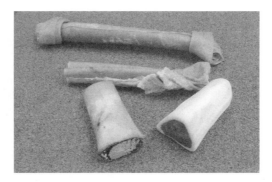

Fig. 14.3 Supplementary foods – chew types for dogs.

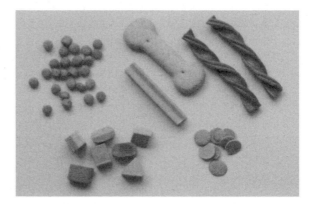

Fig. 14.4 Supplementary foods – biscuit types and shapes.

Meals need to be frequent throughout the day (i.e. a three-month-old puppy needs 4–6 meals), dividing the diet evenly between each one. The stomach size of young animals is too small to cope with only one or two meals a day. By 6 months of age the frequency of meals is usually at 2–3 meals a day, down to 1–2 meals daily by one year of age for a dog. Cats tend to snack as adults and will often stay on 2–3 meals daily.

The above information will vary from animal to animal. Owners generally notice that one of the meals for puppies and kittens is often not eaten, the food in that meal should then be spread through the remaining feeding times until the adult routine is reached.

When adult, usually a pet dog will be fed once or twice daily, a cat will be fed 2–3 meals daily, as required. A lot will depend on the type of food (canned, moist or dry) as to the feeding times, or an unlimited feeding method can be used in cats on dry diets.

Commercial foods are available in formulas for growing puppy and kitten needs. It is important that food chunks are appropriate in size to the animal. Texture is also important: with only milk (or deciduous) teeth, chewing is not possible.

Adult

Once established, feeding routines should not be altered in timing, place or diet types. To do so is stressful to an animal and appetite may decrease as a result. Feeding times should never be too late in the evening, because the animal may need to urinate or defaecate within 3–4 hours of eating, by which time it may be shut in and the owners in bed.

Commercial diets all have information on feeding and quantities, but if part of the ration is always left uneaten, reduce the amount of food until all is eaten at each meal. To maintain the animal's interest, many owners supplement the diet with meal scrapes, gravy, etc. Cat foods are produced in many flavours, some owners using a different one for each day of the week. The condition, energy levels, health status and body weight of the animal need to be monitored to ensure that the diet suits the individual animal. If any change in the diet is considered, always introduce the new diet slowly over a number of days, overlapping it with the old diet to avoid any gut upset.

Working dogs

Depending on the training, working, resting times and function, working dogs may need quite different diets and feeding routines.

A working dog that runs long distances each day may need as much as 2–3 times the normal recommended adult ration of food, e.g. sheep dogs who may run more than 20 miles a day.

Generally diets are grouped for carbohydrate or fat requirement. Carbohydrates (i.e. cereals as biscuits) release sugars and are useful for dogs that require energy for short duration, i.e. agility dogs, both in practice and competition. Other working breeds that are active for long periods and in all weather conditions will need more energy for running and to hold the body temperature in extreme cold (sheep dogs and sledge dogs). Fat increase in the diet is ideal for these dogs. Protein in increased amounts may be useful for muscle development, but the energy requirements will come from carbohydrate and fat. Diets that have increased carbohydrate and fat levels are often referred to as 'active diets'.

Working dogs are normally fed only a small meal before work, leaving the main meal of two-thirds of the required daily intake to be fed after a rest period, allowing time for proper digestion.

Senior dog and cat

Older animals will vary in condition and health status considerably. There are many commercial diets on the market to choose from. Depending on the health of the animal, some are for use with specific medical diseases, others are more generally restrictive of some nutrients for cases of obesity. These obesity diets are often referred to as 'light diets or reducing diets'.

Older animals may have sight, taste and smell losses, as well as poor appetite, poor teeth and gum condition, all making eating difficult. Many also have reduced movement of food in the gut, leading to constipation problems.

To provide for the nutritional needs of these senior animals, consider:

- Improving the taste/smell of the food by warming it to body temperature
- Using one of the appropriate senior diets on the market (seek veterinary advice first)
- Increased fibre in the diet to prevent constipation, i.e. use of bran
- Use of easily digested high-quality proteins, such as fish, poultry and egg, in the diet base
- Encouraging the animal to eat the daily ration by hand feeding initially
- Feeding small meals throughout the day (up to six), in order for the animal to eat the whole daily ration

Caring for the teeth to encourage eating by preventing the build-up of tartar on the teeth, also check for loss of, or loose, teeth, gum disease and inflammation. All these will affect the animal's ability to eat. Many dogs and cats will allow the owner to clean their teeth with a soft toothbrush or finger brush, but if this is not possible, a teeth de-scale and/or teeth removal by a veterinary surgeon may be required.

Mobility problems and joint disease, in dogs particularly, may make bending to the food and water bowls difficult or impossible. To assist the animal, raise the food and water bowls off the floor on to a low box (Fig. 14.5) with a ridge around the edge (to prevent the bowls falling off). These can be home-made or bought from most pet shops (Fig. 14.6).

Pregnancy

Dog

For most of the pregnancy it is not necessary to increase the quantity of food, provided a balanced, good-quality food product is being used.

It is only during the final three weeks of pregnancy that an increase in food intake is required. This is at the time of most weight gain and growth occurring in the fetuses. Overfeeding before this stage of pregnancy may lead to fat deposits; weight gain as a result may lead to problems during parturition (birthing).

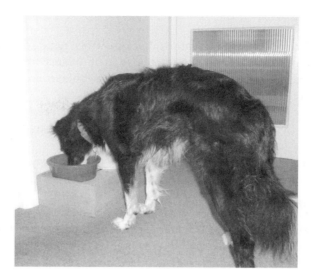

Fig. 14.5 Food bowls on a low box.

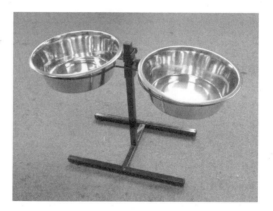

Fig. 14.6 Raised bowl system that can be bought from pet shops.

- Increase food by 10–15% per week from six weeks of pregnancy until parturition. This increases total food intake to approximately 50% over maintenance levels of food being fed
- Use diets formulated for pregnancy and lactation needs
- Feed small meals and often in the final two weeks of pregnancy, to assist food intake
- Provide fresh drinking water, which is always available

Cat

From the time of mating, diet quantities need to be increased for the pregnant cat to approximately 30% above maintenance amounts. Cats will rarely overeat, therefore food can be constantly available as requirements increase.

- Feed a diet formulated for a cat during pregnancy and lactation
- Ensure food is always available (referred to as free-choice feeding), this will help the cat to eat sufficient nutrients
- Provide fresh drinking water, which is always available

How much should be fed?

Amount is based on energy needs and the rate of conversion of food to energy (metabolism) by the individual animal.

Take the number of kcal (kilocalories) of energy needed by an animal and refer to the content tables on any pre-packed food. The manufacturer will use the kcal/day requirements to suggest the amount in weight (grams) of the diet to feed with regard to the percentage value of nutrients in that food.

As a general guide for dogs:

- Small: 250–750 kcal/day
- Medium: 1000–2000 kcal/day
- Large: 2000–2500 kcal/day

Chapter 15
Handling

It is necessary to appreciate the behavioural differences between species in order to perform handling safely. Body language is quite complex in some species, i.e. the dog, and must be taken into account before approaching.

Handling may give rise to fear and stress in the animal, which may be a learned response after a bad handling experience. Any knowledge of the individual's temperament or behaviour in given situations and previous required handling is helpful information.

Reasons for handling

- Daily and weekly checks
- Grooming
- Transportation
- First aid situation
- Examination after injury
- Medicating

Animals should be accustomed to handling from an early age. Teaching the animal to tolerate having difficult areas, such as ears, feet and mouth, looked at will make life less stressful for animal and handler at a later date.

Approaching to handle

- Assess animal's behaviour and body language.
- Be quiet but confident to establish dominance of the situation.
- Talk in a reassuring manner.
- Never corner the animal; always leave supposed choices.
- With a dog or cat, reach out to introduce yourself to the animal.
- Stroke the animal and accustom it to voice and scent.
- Only lift the animal if the approach has been accepted.
- Handle with minimum restraint, especially cats.
- If the animal becomes or is aggressive, then a firm method of restraint is needed for the safety of handlers.

Behaviour seen when animals are unwilling to be handled

- *Cats* – hiss, adopt defensive posture, growl, strike with front claws and flatten their ears to the skull.
- *Dogs* – hackles raised, growling, lips in snarl position, ears forward, barking and attempting to bite.
- *Rabbits* – biting, scratching using hind legs, thumping hind legs on floor and, if terrified, squealing.
- *Guinea pigs* – are not aggressive but will stampede or circle their housing in an effort to get away.
- *Rats* – bite if startled or hurt.

Holding procedures

Rat

Place hand firmly over back and rib cage, restrain head with thumb and forefinger immediately behind lower jaw (Figs 15.1 and 15.2).

Guinea pig

Grasp under the trunk with one hand while supporting the hindquarters with the other hand (Fig. 15.3).

Gerbil

Never lift by the middle or end of the tail. The tail is firmly grasped at the base and the gerbil is lifted and cradled in the palm of the hand. Use the over-the-back grip to prevent struggling (Figs 15.4 and 15.5).

Rabbit

Never lift using only the ears.

- *Short distances* (for cleaning housing) – grasp the skin over the neck with one hand and support the hindquarters with the other (Fig. 15.6).
- *Longer distances* – having lifted the rabbit from housing using the above method, it is positioned against the handler with its head tucked under the handler's arm, the hindquarters being supported by the handler's arms (Fig. 15.7).

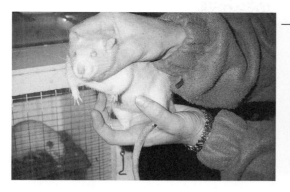

Fig. 15.1 Correct holding technique for a rat.

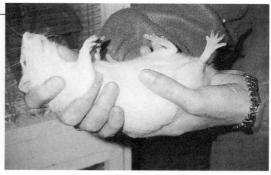

Fig. 15.2 Correct holding technique to expose the abdomen and chest.

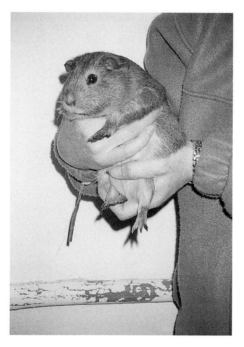

Fig. 15.3 Holding technique for a guinea pig.

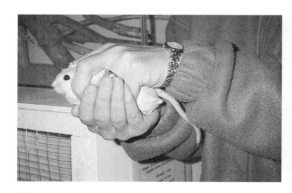

Fig. 15.4 Holding a gerbil.

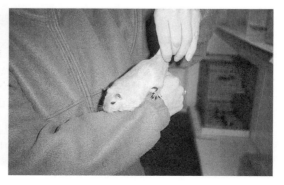

Fig. 15.5 Restraint for a gerbil.

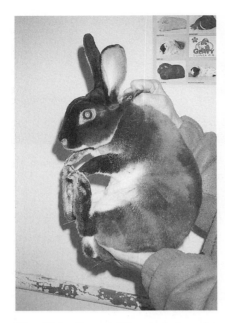

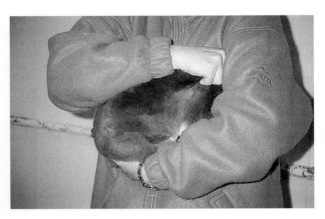

Fig. 15.7 Correct technique for moving a rabbit longer distances.

Fig. 15.6 Correct lifting technique for rabbits.

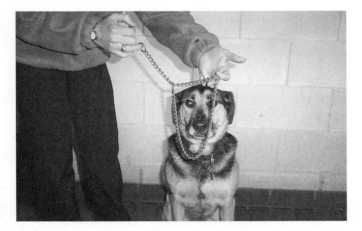

Fig. 15.8 Check chain position – correct size and correctly held.

Dog

Before handling, always check the following:

- The collar is correctly fitted and will not slip off.
- Position of check chain (correct size/correct fit) (Fig. 15.8).
- Temperament (muzzle if necessary).
- Reason for handling.

To tape muzzle a dog

Two handlers are required, one to hold the dog and one to apply the muzzle.

Dog handler

*   Stands facing the same way as the dog and to one side (alongside the shoulder).
*   Takes hold of the scruff and collar (if worn) with both hands, behind the dog's ears.

Person applying tape muzzle

*   Use a bandage which will not stretch.
*   Cut a length in excess to requirements.
*   Make a loop with a double throw knot (Fig. 15.9).

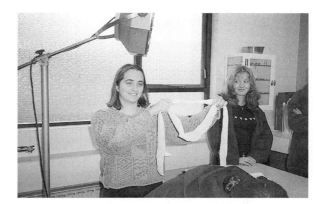

Fig. 15.9   Make a loop with the tape muzzle, with a double throw knot.

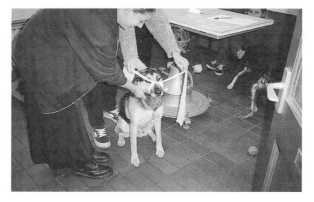

Fig. 15.10   Drop the loop over the dog's mouth and nose and tighten the loop.

Continued

To tape muzzle a dog (*Continued*)

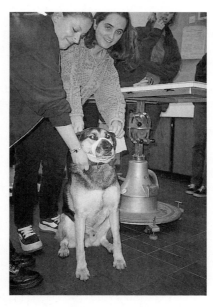

Fig. 15.11   Knot the ends behind the ears and tie a bow for quick release.

- Keeping the loop open, approach from the side of the dog.
- Drop the loop over the dog's mouth and nose and tighten the loop quickly (Fig. 15.10).
- Cross the muzzle ties under the jaw.
- Knot the ends behind the dog's ears and tie into a bow for quick release (Fig. 15.11).

Restraint procedures in the dog and cat

For intravenous injection

Presenting one of the forelegs for procedures such as an injection into the vein or taking a blood sample (Figs 15.12, 15.13 and 15.14).

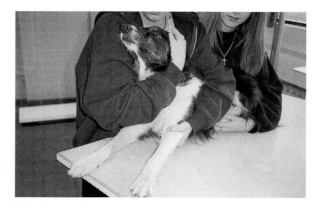

Fig. 15.12 Position for i.v. restraint.

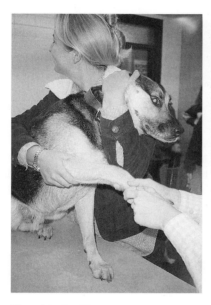

Fig. 15.13 Place thumb over the upper part of the leg and rotate the vein from medial to cranial surface.

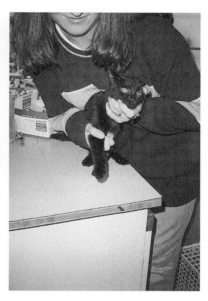

Fig. 15.14 Restraint by one person of a cat for i.v.

For subcutaneous injection

Using the scruff area on the back of the neck (Figs 15.15 and 15.16).

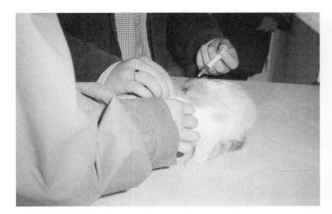

Fig. 15.15 Cat in sitting position.

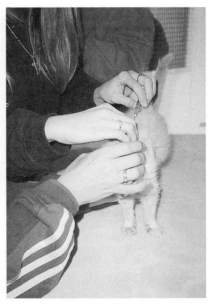

Fig. 15.16 Cat in standing position.

For intramuscular injection

Using the muscle on the front of the hind leg. Never use the muscle at the back (caudal aspect) of the hind leg, to prevent damage to the main nerve supply (sciatic nerve). Two handlers are required, one to control the head and one to give the injection (Fig. 15.17).

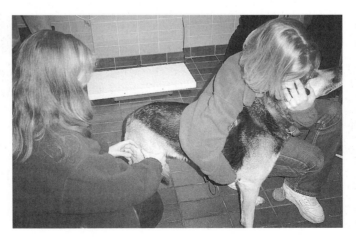

Fig. 15.17 Dog standing – restraint for injection into the front/cranial part of the upper hind leg.

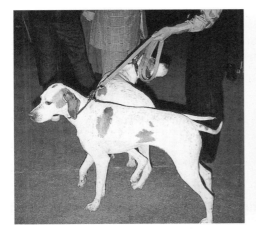

Fig. 16.1   Smooth coat – Pointer.

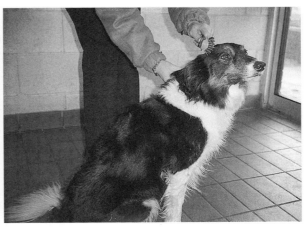

Fig. 16.2   Double coat – Collie.

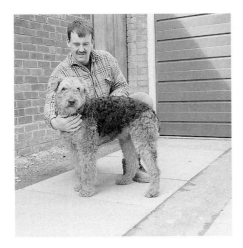

Fig. 16.3   Wire coat – Airedale.

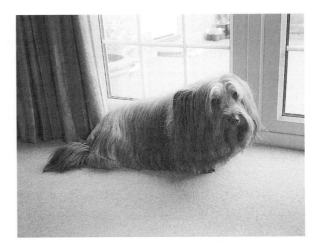

Fig. 16.4   Silky coat – Skye Terrier.

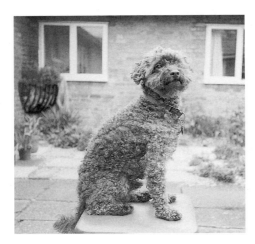

Fig. 16.5   Woolly/curly coat – Poodle.

Environmental temperature

Dogs kept in centrally heated housing will shed their coat continuously. Dogs kept in outside kennels will shed in spring and autumn.

Ill health

If the animal becomes debilitated due to acute or chronic illness the coat growth cycle will be interrupted.

Diet

A balanced diet with all essential nutrients will ensure normal coat growth and condition.

Hormone levels

Levels will alter during oestrus in the bitch, slowing the rate of growth. The coat texture can alter in some disease conditions which affect the body's hormone levels, not only causing the coat to grow more slowly but also making it coarse and rough to touch.

Grooming notes

Smooth coat

Matting of this type of coat does not occur due to its short length. However, the coat will become clogged with dead hair when moulting. Increased grooming at this time will keep the skin in good condition. To prevent loss of natural oils in the coat, only bath if really necessary. If the coat is muddy, brush it out once the coat is dry.

    Equipment required:

- *Short coat* – use a hound glove
- *Long coat* – use a comb and a bristle brush

Double coat

Will matt and tangle if not groomed frequently. Regular grooming sessions of up to three-quarters of an hour to one hour may be necessary to prevent the coat tangling. Some breeds in this category, for example the Old English Sheepdog, are clipped to about 2.5 cm in length in order to simplify grooming. This summer clip will allow the dog to cope better in hot weather.

Bath only 3–4 times yearly, preferably twice yearly, in spring and autumn to condition the coat and clean the skin. Brush out mud once dry and regularly comb out the undercoat during the moulting season.

Equipment required:

- Bristle brush
- Slicker/carder brush
- Comb

Wiry coat

To avoid matting of the coat, these breeds need regular combing. Their top coat is stripped and plucked or machine clipped at three-monthly intervals, followed by a bath to condition and clean the skin. Should mats occur, work them out carefully with the correct dematting equipment.

Equipment required:

- Slicker/carder brush
- Comb
- Dematting comb

Silky coat

Without frequent attention, these coats become very tangled. The coat is so fine in these breeds that it is hard to untangle even with dematting combs. Spaniels and Afghan hounds must have the dead coat hair stripped out every 3–4 months. At this time the coat is usually trimmed, paying particular attention to ears and feet. The fine hair in the ear canals should be plucked at regular intervals and the foot hair trimmed to reduce mud and the attachment of barbed grass seeds.

Bath as required to help both grooming and skin condition using a frequent-use shampoo.

Equipment required:

- Bristle brush
- Dematting comb
- Slicker brush

Woolly/curly coat

Frequently referred to as the non-shedding coat, which does not moult but which grows continuously. As a result of this growth, these breeds need clipping followed by bathing every 6–8 weeks. If not groomed out, the dead hair will form a felt-like mass. The ear canals need constant plucking to prevent these mats which soon plug with ear wax and may lead to infection if not attended to.

Equipment required:

- Comb
- Slicker/carder brush
- Dematting comb
- Scissors

Grooming equipment

Every dog needs its own grooming equipment, normally bought when setting up a new puppy. Equipment to choose from includes the following:

- Brushes:
  - (a) bristle brush
  - (b) slicker/carder brush
  - (c) hound glove
  - (d) rubber brush.
- Combs:
  - (a) fine comb
  - (b) wide-toothed comb
  - (c) rake comb
  - (d) flea/louse comb
  - (e) dematting comb.
- Cutting equipment:
  - (a) stripping knife or comb
  - (b) thinning scissors
  - (c) scissors
  - (d) electric clippers
  - (e) nail clippers.

Brushes

Bristle brushes are available in a range of sizes and shapes. The handle is made of either wood or rigid plastic, with synthetic or natural bristles. The bristles are set close together, making this an ideal surface-only brush. It is unable to penetrate dense coats but is ideal for smooth coats and the removal of mud or other surface material stuck to the hair. On short smooth coats, it can be used with pressure on areas of the dog's back, flanks and hindquarters. The main effect of this surface brushing is to stimulate the skin and distribute the natural oils from the skin to the hair shaft ends, giving a shine to the coat.

Pin brushes are also available in a range of sizes. The handle is made of either wood or a rigid plastic. The pins, often with plastic-coated tips to prevent scratch-

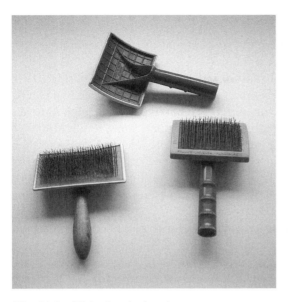

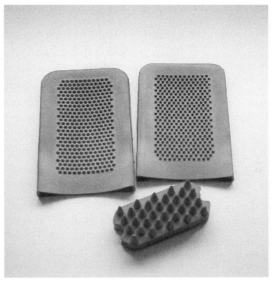

Fig. 16.6 Slicker/carder brushes.

Fig. 16.7 Hound glove (top) and rubber brush (below).

ing the skin surface, are set in a flexible rubber-backed cushion. The pin brush will separate hairs and lay the coat in position, particularly useful for the silky long coats and double coats. These brushes also stimulate the skin, distributing the natural oils from the skin to the tips of the hairs. If the coat has tangled hair or knots, then use a comb first to remove these before brushing. This will prevent the coat being pulled or broken when the pin brush is used.

Slicker/carder brushes (Fig. 16.6), with a wooden or rigid plastic handle, come in a range of sizes. The pins are hooked and set in a rubber-backed cushion, giving some flexibility to the grooming movement. The function of these hooked pins is to remove dead coat. No pressure should be applied when using the slicker brush because the pins could easily scratch or damage the skin surface. It can be used on a range of coat types from silky to double and in some body areas of curly and wire-coated breeds. Never use on areas of the body where the coat is normally thin such as the stomach, groin or armpits.

A *hound glove* (Fig. 16.7) fits over the groomer's hand like a mitten or glove, as the name suggests. It is made of flexible plastic or rubber with short bristles made from wire or plastic and some have a velvet-type surface on one side and bristles on the other. It is used to remove dead or moulting hair (bristle side) and to polish the coat (velvet side) in smooth and short-coated breeds. Care should be taken when using the bristle side, in case too much pressure is used and the skin is damaged.

Combs

Combs are used to remove dead hair and prevent mats forming behind the ears, in the neck/collar area and over the hindquarters.

Combs are available in metal or plastic, with or without handles (Fig. 16.8). Some combs are half wide toothed and half fine toothed so that each half can be used in different body areas and on different coat types. The teeth tips are rounded or plastic coated to avoid tearing the skin surface. Some combs also have pins set so that they are able to roll individually and prevent coat damage when in contact with a mat or tangle.

Combs should be used carefully, especially when encountering a knot or tangle. Slowly tease the hairs and never rush this stage or the coat will be pulled, hurting the dog and making it unwilling to be groomed.

Rake combs (Fig. 16.9) have ridged metal teeth with round tips, set perpendicular to the handle, and resemble a small garden rake. They should not be used by pressing into the coat. Their function is to break up mats and, in dense coats, lift and remove dead undercoat hair. They are pulled towards the groomer through the coat and in the direction of the coat hair.

Flea combs have fine teeth set close together, with a grip area. These are pulled slowly and carefully through the coat, going with the normal coat direction. If a parasite is encountered, the gap between the teeth is too small for it to pass through so it is lifted onto the comb for the groomer to remove.

Dematting combs (Fig. 16.10) have wooden handles and teeth which on one side are rounded and blunt and on the other side are a series of cutting blades. These combs are used, with extreme care, to cut through large mats of hair by placing the blunt side against the dog's skin surface and with a gentle sawing action cutting away from the skin surface and through the mat. This will allow the matted areas to either be combed out or further subdivided for combing and removal of the dead hair.

Cutting equipment

A *stripping knife or comb* (Fig. 16.11) is used to remove dead hair and at the same time trim the live hair. The comb has a serrated metal cutting edge, set against a guard plate on one side for the removal of dead hair. The stripping knife has a metal handle and blade. Sections of coat hair are held between the operator's thumb and the blade and the blade is pulled away from the skin with a twisting movement. At the same time, dead hair can be pulled or plucked. This is known as hand stripping and is used on wire-coated breeds such as terriers, wire-coated Dachshunds and Schnauzers. If done correctly, it is not at all painful.

Thinning scissors (Fig. 16.12) have one regular and one serrated blade or both blades serrated. They thin the coat without affecting its appearance. These scissors are therefore used on the undercoat, preserving the colour of the outer coat appearance.

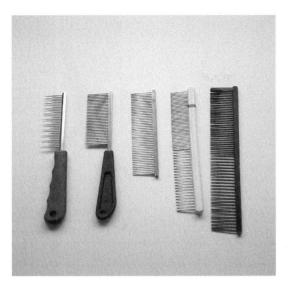

Fig. 16.8   Comb types.

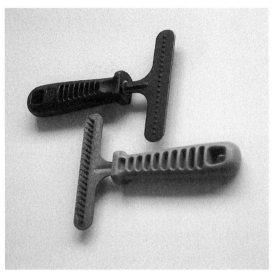

Fig. 16.9   Rake comb.

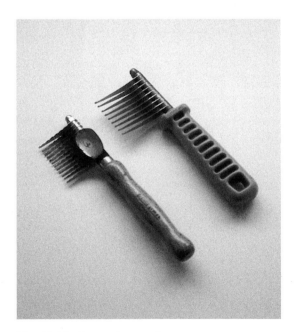

Fig. 16.10   Dematting comb.

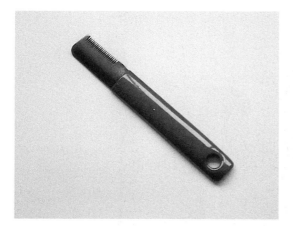

Fig. 16.11 Stripping knife.

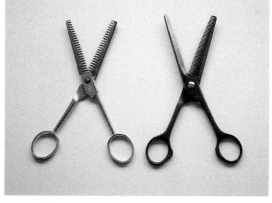

Fig. 16.12 Thinning scissors or shears.

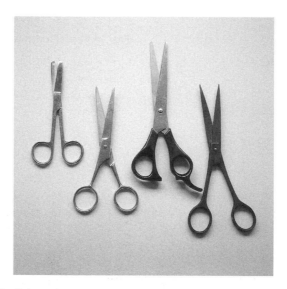

Fig. 16.13 Scissor types.

Scissors (Fig. 16.13) are available in many sizes and shapes for use on the various body areas, from long, sharp, tapering blades to short, blunt-ended blades, depending on the area that requires a trim. Blunt-ended scissors are used to trim between toes and in delicate areas around the eyes, ears, lips and genitals.

Electric clippers (Fig. 16.14) are used by professional groomers in conjunction with scissors, particularly in the curly-coated breeds such as the poodle. These coats keep growing all year round and need constant attention. Always keep the blade of the clippers flat to the coat to avoid cutting the skin.

The clipper cuts away the excess hair more rapidly than scissors and is used with a variety of detachable blades. The blades vary from fine tooth for close

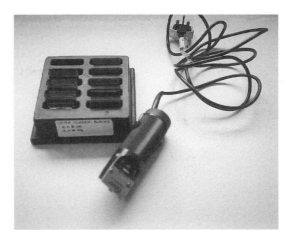

Fig. 16.14 Electric clipper with range of blades.

trims to ones set with wide-spaced blades or teeth, which leave short hairs against the skin surface. The blades are snapped onto a post on the clipper only when the clipper is running.

The clipper is held like a pencil which gives a firm grip, allowing the groomer to move over the coat lightly and keep the blade flat against the section being clipped.

Clippers will get hot during use so it is important to closely monitor the blade temperature in order to prevent a clipper burn or rash developing on the damaged skin surface. There are several ways of avoiding this:

- Spray hot blades with aerosol lubricant spray to reduce temperature.
- Change the hot blade for a new cool blade.
- Use a second clipper, allowing the first to cool.
- Keep the blades in use sharpened.
- Only clip hair that is completely dry.

Nail clippers (Fig. 16.15) are only used to cut nails which are overlong. A range of clippers is available, from the guillotine clipper (also useful in small mammals) to the double blade type. The choice of nail clipper will depend on the length and position of the nail presented.

Grooming procedure

Depending on the coat type of a dog, grooming will be a daily and/or a weekly event. It provides the owner with the opportunity not only to condition the coat and skin but to:

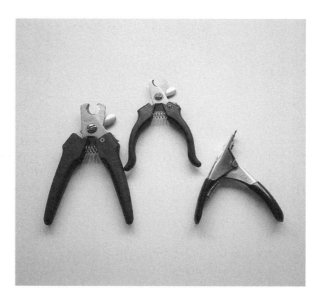

Fig. 16.15 Types of nail clippers.

- Clean any discharge and examine the eyes
- Check and clean the ear to prevent infection developing
- Clean and examine the mouth and particularly the teeth
- Examine and trim any overlong toe nails
- Check the anal region

Eyes should be bright and free of any discharge. If any discharge is seen in the corner of the eye, moisten a clean piece of cotton wool with water and wipe away in the direction of the nose. If the discharge looks anything other than clear, check for signs of inflammation and seek veterinary attention.

Ears should be free of wax, a dull pink colour and without odour. In the curly-coated breeds, the ears need to be plucked free of hair which, if left in place, attracts wax, parasites and infection. Check for signs of discomfort or reluctance by the dog when the flap is being examined, which may indicate a problem.

Mouth. The gums and tongue should be pink (pigmented in the Chow chow) or partly pink with pigmented areas. Gums should be well defined around each tooth, with no food or other materials attached. In order to prevent any build-up of tartar on the teeth, pet toothpaste in various flavours and tooth brushes can be used as part of the daily grooming examination.

Feet or paws should be clean around the nail bed, nails just in contact with the ground, excess hair cut short between the pads and nails to prevent mats and grass seed barbs penetrating the skin and causing an abscess.

Anal region under the tail and around the anus needs to be checked daily in dogs, whether short or long coated. The area should be free of any faecal material and show no signs of redness or inflammation. Should the dog start

between the owner and the animal. This attention is particularly important if the kitten is to be a show animal.

Cats spend a considerable part of every day in self-grooming. They have a specially adapted tongue with backward-facing barbs for the removal of dead hairs from the coat.

Grooming will:

- Remove dead hair
- Remove material from coat surface
- Stimulate skin and distribute secreted oils for coat condition
- Provide a feeling of well-being

Constant grooming in long-haired cats can cause health problems. During self-grooming the cat will swallow large quantities of saliva and wet hair, which forms *hair balls* or sausage-shaped plugs in the stomach. This ingested hair can cause an obstruction in the digestive tract.

In the event of loss of appetite, weight loss or constipation, contact a veterinary surgeon for advice.

The coat

Selective breeding and genetic mutation have enhanced cats' coats or caused coat loss. The cat has a top coat of *guard hair* and an undercoat which consists of coarse, bristly *awn* hairs and soft downy hairs.

Examples of coat type are as follows:

- *Short hair*, e.g. British short hair, has short guard hairs with even shorter but slightly curly awn hairs as a sparse undercoat.
- *Long hair*, e.g. Persian, has extremely long guard hairs with a thick undercoat of downy hair which gives this breed its full, dense coat.
- *Curly coat*, e.g. Cornish Rex, has very short curly awn and downy hairs of the same length and no guard hairs at all.
- *Wire hair*, e.g. American wire hair, has short curly, even coiled guard hairs, down and awn.
- *Hairless*, e.g. Sphinx, which has a coat so sparse as to appear hairless but in fact has a covering of downy hairs on the legs, tail and face only.

The cat has three kinds of skin gland to care for its coat. Two types are sweat-producing glands, some located only on the pads of the feet, others over the entire body used to leave its scent and mark territory. Territory marking is seen when the cat rubs against objects. The third type of gland is the sebaceous gland near the hair follicles which secretes sebum to help waterproof the coat.

Moulting occurs in the spring and autumn, when the coat comes out in what seem like handfulls at a time. Long-haired coats moult all year round due to the constant room temperatures in which these cats tend to live. It is therefore essential that the long-coated breeds have owners who realise the necessity of daily grooming routines.

Grooming notes

Short coat

These cats are efficient self-groomers, with the normal-shaped head giving a slightly longer tongue than in the long-coated breeds. Two half-hour grooming sessions per week are ideal. In between, continue to condition the coat by stroking along the lie of the hair or polishing the coat using a piece of silk, velvet or chamois leather cloth.

Equipment required:

- Fine-toothed comb
- Soft bristle brush
- Rubber brush (see Fig. 16.7)
- Chamois cloth

Long coat

With the shorter faces resulting in shorter tongues, these breeds tend to be less efficient groomers. Moulting all year round, the coat tends to mat. Grooming is needed daily, split into two half-hour sessions during the day to check for mats. Start with a normal comb to remove dead hair and then use a fine comb to fluff up the coat. A toothbrush is used to brush the face hair, keeping well clear of the eyes.

Equipment required:

- Wide-toothed and fine-toothed combs
- Slicker brush
- Bristle brush
- Toothbrush – medium bristle

Curly coat

Should not be overgroomed as this could result in baldness. A soft brush with short bristles is sufficient for removal of dead coat. Groom twice weekly.

Equipment required:

- Soft bristle brush

Wire coat

These have a crimped, woolly coat which is coarse to the touch. Removal of the dead hair is essential but ensure that the curls spring untangled back into position. This is achieved by minimum brushing with a soft bristle brush and hand stroking at least twice weekly.

Equipment required:

• Soft bristle brush

Hairless coat

With hair only on extremities, skin conditioning is more essential. Do not brush these breeds. The skin needs daily sponging to remove *dander* (small scales from the hair and dried skin secretions). A sponge moistened with warm water wiped over the body daily or more frequently if required will remove the dander which, if left, could cause a skin allergy.

Equipment required:

• Sponge

Bathing

Groom out all mats and hair contaminated with faeces. If these mats cannot be groomed out, it may be necessary to cut them off with scissors.

As with the dog, make sure all equipment is to hand before starting. A non-slip surface in the bath is essential in order to give the cat something to cling to. Unless bathing is a routine experience, cats can find it very traumatic so only bath if really necessary.

Two people are required, one to hold and reassure, one to bath.

• Fill the bath with about 10 cm of warm water into which the cat is lowered gently.
• A mixer hose and/or a sponge are used to soak the coat hair and apply the shampoo. Proceed with a thorough rinse and then wrap the cat in a towel.
• At all times, make sure water or shampoo never gets close to the eyes, ears or mouth.
• Wipe over the face with cotton wool moistened in warm water.
• Towel dry and keep in a warm area until fully dry.
• If the cat will tolerate it, use an electric dryer set only to warm and held at a safe distance.
• Once the coat is dry, comb out gently and brush.

Finish with the grooming of the coat hair.

- *Short hair* – start at the head and comb/brush towards the tail, including chest and abdomen. Then rub down with a chamois or nylon pad to polish the coat.
- *Long hair* – comb legs free of tangles then abdomen, flanks, back, chest and neck, then the tail section, fluffing out the coat hair by brushing the wrong way. Finally, using a toothbrush, groom the face hair.

When all grooming is complete, remove the dead hair from the combs and brushes, wash, disinfect and rinse before storing to prevent cross infection between grooming sessions or infecting another animal groomed with the same equipment.

Warning

If the coat is dirtied by chemicals such as tar, creosote, paint or oil, remove as soon as possible to prevent absorption through the skin or self-grooming and ingestion of the chemical, which may be a poison. Never use chemicals to remove these substances. On a dry coat, use soft margarine, washing-up liquid or liquid paraffin to work the substance free of the hairs, then proceed with a bath and dry thoroughly. If the cat has self-groomed, contact a veterinary surgeon immediately for advice.

Chapter 17
Pets: Mammals, Birds and Fish

General husbandry for mammals and birds

Small mammals may not be used to handling and can bite. Initial restraint should be firm but gentle to prevent injury (Fig. 17.1).

Housing

Cages, runs, housing and pens need to be well made and of materials suitable to the species being housed. To prevent injury, housing should:

- Have no sharp edges
- Have no rough surfaces
- Be in good repair
- Be easy to clean
- Be escape proof
- Be large enough for free movement and exercise
- Be dry and well ventilated
- Be heated or cooled as required during the seasonal changes in environmental temperature
- Have a supply of electricity
- Have no direct sunlight into housing
- Not be subject to temperature extremes

Health

A regular examination to determine health status or detect injury is required. If any animal is found to be diseased, it is important to move it to isolation or quarantine areas.

Only purchase animals from a reputable and reliable source. It is easy to introduce disease to an animal collection, which can be hard to treat and eliminate.

To maintain health:

- Clean housing thoroughly
- Move any sick animal to isolation
- Apply high levels of hygiene to all equipment

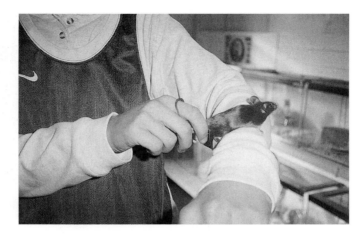

Fig. 17.1   Gentle restraint, allowing the mouse to explore without escaping.

- Have a good air flow through the housing to prevent breathing problems and airborne diseases
- House different species separately where possible
- Change bedding several times a week, depending on species

Nutrition

The needs of each species of animal have been well documented. However, there are general guidelines:

- Feed only fresh and clean leafy foods
- Check that the feed container is in date, has not been broken open or damaged and is not contaminated
- Feed must provide all the nutrients necessary for full health
- Water is fresh and always available
- Water containers/feeders are cleaned regularly
- Food is stored in closed containers at room temperature and kept dry

MAMMALS

Rabbits

There are over 80 breeds of rabbit, with variation in shape, colour, size and character. Belonging to the order Lagomorpha, they usually fall into three main categories:

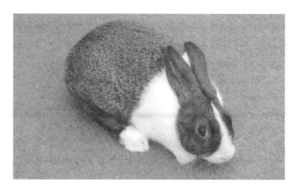

Fig. 17.2   Dutch rabbit (short coated).

- *Normal* – these breeds have a coat type of short, dense fur, similar to that of the wild rabbit, and were bred originally for meat, e.g. New Zealand White, Chinchilla, Dutch (Fig. 17.2) and Californian
- *Fancy* – mainly bred for show, with distinguishing features, e.g. Lop for their large ears, Netherland Dwarf and Flemish Giant for their size, Himalayan for their coat markings
- *Rex and Satin* – noted for their velvet- or satin-like coats in which the guard hairs are missing, or below the under-hair level, giving the coat a smooth, dense appearance

Rabbits are social animals and should not be kept on their own. In the wild they live in groups with a well-defined hierarchy. The males will fight to defend territory if kept in the same housing, as they would in the wild. Females will live together happily, but are likely to show dominant aggression once maturity is reached. Most owners pair up male and female, with one or both neutered if not intending to breed from them. Sometimes rabbits can be paired with other species, such as guinea-pigs, but this is not always ideal because the rabbits do tend to bully the guinea-pig (being a smaller animal), also the two species have different nutritional requirements, making feeding difficult. A rabbit kept alone needs a lot of human interaction to prevent fear or aggressive behaviour. To enable this, some single rabbits are trained to use litter trays and are kept as house pets.

Biological data

Male	buck
Female	doe
Offspring	kits (kittens)
Adult weight	1–10 kg (depending on breed)
Maturity	12 weeks onwards

Continued

Guinea-pigs

Guinea-pigs (*Cavia aperea porcellus*) are also known as 'cavies', belonging to the order Rodentia under the suborder Hystricomorphs, which includes chinchillas. There are three main coat types of guinea-pig, within which there are many colour and marking variations. These can be grouped as:

- Smooth or short hair (also referred to as self varieties), e.g. Self Golden or Dutch
- Containing whirls, ridges and rosettes, e.g. Abyssinian
- Long coated (up to 50 cm in length) with long, straight hairs, e.g. Peruvian and Sheltie. This type requires a lot of grooming and is mostly kept for showing, therefore not recommended for beginners

Guinea-pigs are nervous animals but are popular as pets. They are generally docile, rarely biting, and are easy to handle and tame. They should not be kept on their own because they are very sociable animals. All-female or all-male groups can live together; however, the males must not be housed anywhere near the females as once they are sexually mature they will fight for dominance. Females and males can be neutered if non-breeding mixed groups are to be kept as pets.

Guinea-pigs are not as agile as many of the other rodents, but although they have short legs and stocky bodies, they are able to run quite quickly, especially when startled. For communication they are capable of making a range of noises, from squeaks and squeals to grunts. Although guinea-pigs do not dig, they are at home in dense undergrowth, and enjoy making 'runs' through long grass. The main difference between the cavy and other rodents is the length of gestation and the resulting advanced stage of their young at birth.

Biological data

Male	boar
Female	sow
Offspring	piglets
Adult weight	75–100 g
Maturity	males: 8–10 weeks
	females: 4–5 weeks
Gestation period	60–72 days
Litter size	2–6 (average size)
Weaning age	3–4 weeks
Body temperature	38–39°C
Life span	4–7 years

Anatomical facts

Teeth

Dental formula: incisors 1/1; canines 0/0 (diastema); premolars 1/1; molars 3/3.

The teeth are open rooted and chisel shaped, continuing to grow throughout the guinea-pig's lifetime. Guinea-pigs do not have the second small pair of incisors (peg teeth) found behind the main pair in rabbits; however, they do have the gap behind the incisors called the diastema. This allows the sides of the cheeks to be drawn in behind the incisors, enabling the animal to continue gnawing while regulating what it swallows.

Tail

Born without a tail.

Scent glands

Sebaceous glands are located on the rump and used to mark territory.

Pelvis

The pubic symphysis (floor of the pelvic joint) will separate under the influence of hormones during parturition, in order to allow the newborn passage through the birth canal. Newborn guinea-pigs are referred to as *precocious*, meaning that within a few hours of birth they are self-sufficient, eating and drinking from feeding dishes. They are born with a complete coat, eyes and ears open, and with a set of teeth in place.

Housing

Guinea-pigs are sociable and can be housed as a colony. A single animal can be housed with another species such as a rabbit breed of similar size (see Fig. 17.4).

Housing should:

- Protect from extremes of temperature in summer and winter, similar to the rabbit
- Protect the animal from getting wet and exposure to draughts
- Be well constructed from good-quality materials which have not been treated with any toxic chemicals
- Be the correct size; rabbit housing can accommodate 2–3 guinea-pigs
- Provide good air flow and ventilation
- Have a summer run for natural grazing, or wire off a part of the garden to allow for space and freedom to exercise

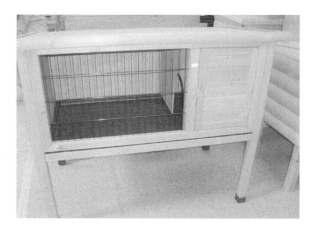

Fig. 17.5 Type of hutch used in housing.

- Be easy to clean. Use similar bedding as that used for rabbits, but it must be clean, dry and dust free. Guinea-pigs tend not to toilet in one area, so more frequent cleaning is required than for the rabbit. If feeding and water bowls are used, these need daily washing as they tend to be fouled.

An example of guinea-pig housing is shown in Fig. 17.5.

Food and water

Guinea-pigs often chew feed and water containers. Choose a suitable indestructible material.

Guinea-pigs are herbivores and spend most waking hours grazing if allowed. By nature, guinea-pigs dislike any change to their routines, so watch for correct use of water feeders, if any changes have been made to equipment.

Commercially available pelleted guinea-pig feed can be used. If any other prepared diet is used, then it is essential to supplement vitamin C, as ascorbic acid, in the diet, for skin and coat condition. Guinea-pigs are unable to manufacture vitamin C and must receive a dietary source. Although some vitamin C can be obtained from natural grazing, they must have a daily supply of 10 mg/kg body weight. During pregnancy the quantity of vitamin C must be increased by three times the normal daily amount to maintain a healthy animal.

Some rabbit diets may also contain levels of vitamin D that are too high for the guinea-pig. Read the packaging and ask the supplier for advice. Supply good-quality roughage such as hay or cut grass. Supplement pelleted food with fresh vegetables (swedes and carrots) and fruit. Useful green foods include broccoli, dandelion and groundsel. Always provide fresh drinking water daily, using similar drinking bottles and spouts to those found in rabbit housing.

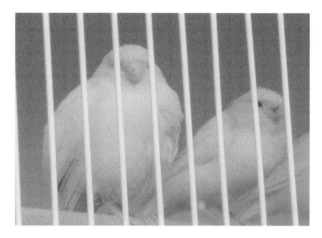

Fig. 17.9 Canaries.

are too rich in fat and calcium, which can lead to dietary imbalance and ill health. An animal protein source may be included in a commercial gerbil food, or table scraps or boiled egg can be added to the diet. Also supplement the diet with fresh fruit and vegetables, such as apple, banana and carrot.

The gerbil will hoard food in a larder area of its housing. Always remove the uneaten food to prevent it becoming stale. Water must be supplied in bottles with sipper tubes, which can be attached to the side of the tank or the lid. The water should be supplied fresh daily.

BIRDS (AVES)

Birds are kept either as pets, for breeding or for exhibition. They can be housed singly in cages of suitable size or in groups in large outdoor aviaries. There are many different species of bird, which are assigned to 27 Orders.

The Orders most commonly seen are:

- Anseriformes – ducks, geese and swans
- Falconiformes – diurnal hawks and falcons
- Galliformes – domestic fowl and pheasants
- Passeriformes – finches and canaries (passerines) (Fig. 17.9)
- Psittiformes – parrots and budgerigars (psittacines)
- Stringiformes – owls
- Clubiformes – pigeons and doves

Most pet cage birds come from one of two main Orders:

- Passerines – perching birds (canary)
- Psittacines – climbing birds (budgerigar)

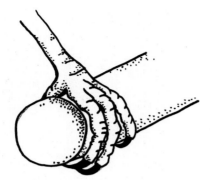

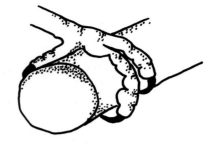

Fig. 17.11   Psittacine foot.

Fig. 17.10   Passerine foot.

The two main features of anatomy which distinguish these two groups are:

- beak conformation – passerines peck at seeds whereas psittacines open fruit and nuts
- feet conformation – passerines have three outer toes facing forward and one inner toe facing backward (Fig. 17.10), whereas psittacines have two middle toes facing forward and two outer toes facing backward (Fig. 17.11)

Other anatomical facts:

- *Skeleton* – bones are thin, some containing air sacs (linked to the respiratory system) making up a lightweight structure for flight.
- *Digestive tract* – food is stored in the crop, the gizzard then grinds the food to pass to the intestines. The opening cloaca is a common end to the outside for the digestive, urinary and reproductive tracts.
- *Respiratory system* – birds have no diaphragm, the lungs are set out in pairs through the thorax and abdomen area (Fig. 17.12). The bird respiratory system is complex for improved flow of air to the tissues.

For many pet owners their choice is the budgerigar. Belonging to the parakeet family of birds, budgerigars have a chattering call and can be taught words and simple tunes. They are easy to keep, both in housing and feeding needs. If let out of their housing into a room, budgerigars will normally return to the accommodation quite readily. Some birds are valued not for their chatter but for their song, such as the canary (particularly the male bird). Canaries belong to the finch family of birds, which are quick moving, hard to catch and usually kept in aviary-type housing and as a group.

If pet birds do share the house un-caged, it is important to remember that birds like to explore and should not be left unattended. Precautions to take before letting the bird out of its cage include:

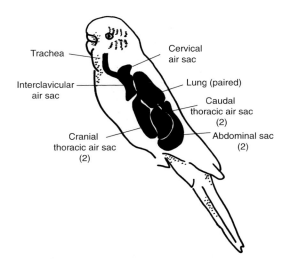

Trachea

Interclavicular air sac

Cranial thoracic air sac (2)

Cervical air sac

Lung (paired)

Caudal thoracic air sac (2)

Abdominal sac (2)

Fig. 17.12 Avian respiratory system.

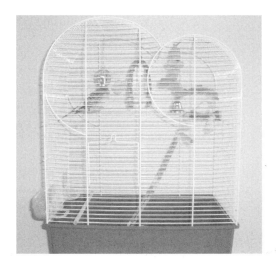

Fig. 17.13 Budgerigar cage type in common use.

- Close all windows and doors
- Do not allow flight or access to the kitchen area, because of hot surfaces and fumes fatal to a bird
- Check that electric cables are not exposed, and that electric fans are switched off
- Remove houseplants that are toxic to birds, such as cacti
- Remove other pets, such as dogs or cats

Housing for pet birds must be cleaned easily, both daily and, more thoroughly, monthly. Birds are kept as pets for many reasons, one of which is to display their beauty, achieved by keeping them in:

- Cages (Fig. 17.13)
- Aviaries

Cage system

There are many types of cage available, with a variety of costs, size and design. However, many are unsuitable for the many varied species kept as pets. A cage should be as large as possible, especially if the bird is going to be confined for much of the day in it.

A cage must:

- Not cause the bird to fly in an artificial way, i.e. circular cages
- Be strong and well constructed with no sharp edges (especially around the cage base)

- Have safe cage fittings, i.e. materials that can not be chewed used for food containers
- Have good door fastenings
- Be easy to keep clean
- Have meshwork or bars on one side to give a feeling of security to the bird
- Be placed well above ground level, i.e. at eye height
- Provide environmental enrichment (toys/activities)
- Have a variety of perches (not covered with sand paper as these can damage feet)
- Be sited away from draughts, direct sunlight and any harmful fumes (cooking fumes, i.e. over-heated oil, cigarette smoke and room sprays)
- Be cleaned daily (removal of unwanted fresh foods, seeds and droppings)

Aviary system

There are many advantages to the pet birds when housed in a larger space such as an aviary. Flight becomes possible, providing a more natural environment, complete with plants and secluded areas. There are disadvantages as well. Aviaries are more difficult to clean, it is more time consuming to remove dropped foods, disease can be carried to the pet birds by wild birds, mice and rats attracted by the uneaten foodstuff. The most obvious concern for birds housed outside is their exposure to cold and hot weather conditions.

An aviary must:

- Be well designed, with a safety door, as large as possible in size, and high enough for good flight but be easy to clean
- Be made of materials that will cause no harm (to include gauge of the netting and wood types used)
- Have a floor/base that is easy to clean, i.e. concrete
- Have perches of different diameters and heights
- Have shallow baths or a misting system for bathing
- Be covered in part (or one entire side), to avoid wind and rain
- Have an inside shelter of boxes to encourage roosting at night
- Ensure a 12-hour period of daylight, using lighting systems in the winter, to encourage food intake in the correct amounts
- Never have food containers placed under perches; preferably they should be off the floor

Budgerigar

The budgerigar is available in a wide range of colours, but in the wild it is green. Belonging to the Order Psittiformes, its species name is *Melopsittacus undulatus*. It originates from the Australian interior, where its natural habitat is semi-arid (hot) grassland with trees, near water holes.

Budgerigars are the most practical of the cage birds. They are lively, colourful, quite hardy, diurnal and can be brought up to mimic human speech. Although they need daily attention, they are reasonably cheap to house and feed.

Biological data

Male	cock
Female	hen
Offspring	chick
Adult weight	30–35 g
Sexing	male bird has blue cere
	female has brown cere
Maturity	5 months onwards
Clutch	3–6 white eggs
Incubation time	18 days to hatch (up to 3 weeks)
Fledgling	further 35 days
Body temperature	40–42°C
Life span	6–8 years

Anatomical fact

Beak

This is a hinge joint between the skull and upper beak. With no teeth, this allows increased movements suitable for slicing through nut shells, with the help of a flexible tongue to obtain food (Fig. 17.14).

Food and water

Budgerigars are fussy and do not like change to their diet. They should be fed a good commercial seed mixture with an iodine supplement (iodine block). Often a combination of canary seed and millet is used in these feeds. A supply of calcium as cuttlefish should be held in the cage clips for the bird to attack.

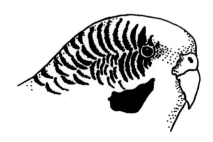

Fig. 17.14   Budgerigar beak.

Fresh fruit, vegetables and green food (dandelion, chickweed, groundsel and lettuce) all add interest and nutrients to the diet.

As seed eaters, budgerigars have evolved to grind seeds in the gizzard using dietary grit. This would be swallowed with food in the wild, but for pet birds this is supplied in soluble form (oyster-shell for minerals) and insoluble form (particles of stone/rock).

Ensure a fresh supply of water, changed daily in the housing (cage or aviary), and thorough cleaning of the water containers to prevent growth of algae.

Canary

The canary is found in a wide range of colours and markings but in the wild is a greenish-yellow colour only. It is part of the finch family of birds, belonging to the Order Passeriformes (passerines). The species title is *Serinus canaria* and it originates from the Canary Islands and parts of Europe.

The natural habitat for the canary is scrubland, fields and pastures, and it is diurnal. Passerines are perching birds, best kept in aviary flocks because it is rare that they are tame enough to handle.

Biological data

Male	cock
Female	hen
Offspring	chick
Adult weight	20 g
Sexing	When mature, both sexes look alike. The male bird song is the best. To be sure of obtaining a male, birds are usually bought several months after fledging, by which time the cock birds will be distinguished by their song
Clutch	3–6 eggs are laid every other day
Incubation time	14 days
Fledgling	further 14 days
Body temperature	40–42°C
Life span	6–9 years

Anatomical fact

Beak

This is short and conical in shape, used to crack seeds when feeding (Fig. 17.15).

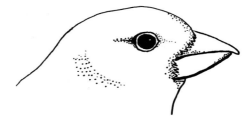

Fig. 17.15   Canary beak.

Food and water

Canaries are hard-billed seed eaters. Their food contains both cereals and oil seeds such as canary seed, millet, rape seed and hemp. It is important to remove the husks from the feed container every day to enable feeding. Appropriately sized grit (soluble and insoluble) must be available in order to grind the seeds in the gizzard.

Commercial complete diets are available, but some fresh green food (lettuce, dandelion, chickweed and alfalfa), fruit and vegetables should also be offered.

Remove any uneaten fresh foods or soaked seeds daily. Soaking enables germination of seeds, which improves the nutritional value, but it is important that these are well drained and removed after a few hours if not eaten, to avoid fungal growth which could be harmful. Tonic foods, which include a greater range of seed types and are for occasional use, are also available commercially.

Ensure a fresh supply of water, changed daily in the housing (cage or aviary), and thorough cleaning of the water containers to prevent growth of algae.

FISH

Fish make excellent pets, they are attractive, colourful, and interesting to study or just watch. Fish do not demand much time and do not make any noise. Feeding costs are low and equipment can be reasonably simple or as elaborate and expensive as you wish to make it.

Types of fish commonly kept as pets fall into three main groups:

- Cold water (10–26°C)
- Tropical freshwater (21–29°C)
- Tropical marine (21–29°C)

Of the three groups, the cold water and tropical freshwater fish are normally kept. Tropical marine fish are complex to keep and a good understanding of their requirements is essential.

Marine fish live in sea water, they are hypotonic (i.e. less salty than the sea water that is their environment); this causes water to be drawn out of these fish

Some fish species in the wild may be found in many continents or only in one lake or river.

Tropical freshwater fish can be divided into two main groups:

- Egg-layer, hatching into fry (i.e. gouramis, tetras, barbs)
- Live-bearer, giving birth to fully formed young which are larger than fry (i.e. platies, guppies)

Coldwater fish

Coldwater fish have a life span of approximately 6–20 years.

Coldwater fish are found in a range of habitats in the wild. The water temperature (10–23°C), the oxygen levels, the speed of the water current and water chemistry will vary depending on location, i.e. lakes, ponds, streams, mountain streams.

The two fish commonly kept from this group are:

- Goldfish
- Koi carp

Goldfish

Goldfish varieties are increasingly diverse as a group.

Ideal conditions:

- Water – neutral pH to slightly alkaline
- Temperature – 10–26°C
- Region – bottom, top and middle

They fall into three main categories:

- Common – the most popular in terms of the number owned; they are a hardy fish, able to live in aquarium or pond
- Single tailed – known for fast swimming ability; the Shubunkin is ideal for a home aquarium, whereas the Comet is better in a pond or large aquarium
- Double tailed – are more unusual and a less hardy type. They are only suitable for deep aquaria and indoor pools. They tend to have a shorter life span due, in part, to their egg-shaped bodies and flotation problems, i.e. Veiltail

Koi carp

Koi carp originated from eastern Asia (Caspian and Aral seas) and China. They are ornamental varieties of the common carp.

Ideal conditions:

- Water – neutral pH, moderately hard
- Temperature – 10–24°C
- Tank region – top, middle and bottom

Koi are messy feeders, requiring a good filtration system to keep the water clear. They tend to destroy plants, therefore the furnishings in an aquarium tend to be bogwood or smooth rock. Koi can be mixed with fancy goldfish if required.

Considerations when setting up an aquarium

Size of aquarium

Standard aquaria can be bought in various combinations of length, width and depth, depending on:

- The species being kept, e.g. the Veiltail goldfish requires a deeper tank because of the size of its double tail
- Stocking density of fish to be kept

Positioning

- Firm foundation – the floor must be able to support the weight of the water-filled tank, ideally over joists not just floor boards
- Away from draughts, heaters and direct sunlight, i.e. not near a window or in a conservatory
- In an area of a room that has no passing traffic
- In a quiet area, too dark for a house plant
- Next to more than one electric socket
- Level the tank and place polystyrene or a foam mat under the tank on the stand, to cushion it from any unevenness in the metalwork of the stand

Substrates

These are materials placed on the bottom of the tank (Fig. 17.17). They include:

- Coarse gravel – best for large tanks; it is used to recreate the bed of a river or stream
- Medium and fine gravel – often mixed and can be used with under-gravel filtration
- Coloured gravel – gaudy but fun; buy from reputable sources to ensure the dyes used are not poisonous

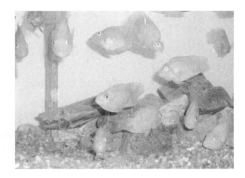

Fig. 17.17   Marine tank substrate.

- Sand – very useful for bottom-dwelling species of fish (there are no sharp points that can injure the fish) and a good substrate for plant growth

Ensure that, whatever the substrate used, it is washed to remove dust particles, dirt and other impurities.

Filter systems

Filter systems are used to clean the water; filtering out wastes such as excess food materials, sections of plants and fish excretions.

- External power filters draw water through the various filter media and pump the clean water back into the tank. These are useful for a smaller aquarium set-up
- Internal power filters also draw water through the various filters but are located inside the tank
- Under-gravel filters consist of one or more perforated plates that cover the base of the aquarium. An air stone or line is attached to a length of tubing and the plates are covered by substrate material. The flow of oxygenated water through the gravel allows filtering

Heating

Heating is used in both coldwater and tropical freshwater tank systems, which require a stable water temperature whatever the environmental temperature may be (even in centrally heated houses, the temperature alters between day and night). Various designs of heater are available (always read the manufacturer's instructions on adjusting the temperature):

- Combined electronic heater/thermostats are located inside the tank (Fig. 17.18)

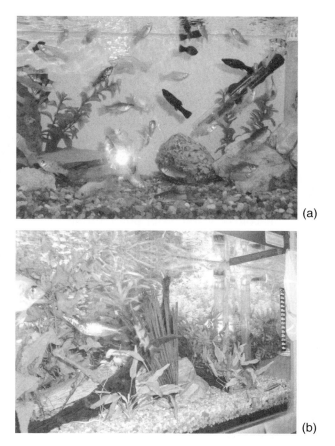
(a)

(b)

Fig. 17.18   (a) Aquarium heater located in the tank. (b) Fish in an established tank.

- Submersible heaters controlled by external or internal thermostats
- Under-tank heating mats controlled by external or internal thermostats

Aquarium hood or cover

- Prevents dust and dirt particles falling into the tank
- Prevents fish escaping
- Keeps out predators such as other household pets
- Helps to retain the tank temperature
- Reduces evaporation

Lighting

Lighting supported in the aquarium hood is essential for the health of the fish and live plants in the tank. Fluorescent tubes have been developed in a number of different colours to imitate daylight, and can be used in combination to show off the fish colours.

Setting up the aquarium

- The aquarium tank is cleaned with dilute detergent to remove any chemicals, rinsed thoroughly and put into position.
- In order to hide the electric cables and filter pipes, choose a decorative plastic background to suit the type of ornament in the tank, the plants and the fish, or have a plain black background. This is a personal choice.
- Next, the filter, substrate (gravel or sand), the heater if required, thermometer, prepared wood, rocks and other furnishings are placed.
- Using cold or warm water poured from a clean measuring jug onto a saucer to prevent disturbance of the substrate gravel, begin to fill the tank. Water can be pre-conditioned by allowing it to stand for several days or by adding a conditioner. This allows evaporation of any chlorine gas.
- If the substrate gravel has been washed properly, there should be little or no clouding of the water as it is added. Once the gravel has been covered, water can be poured in quite quickly to about 10–12 cm from the final water level. Plants (plastic) can be placed when the tank has matured, without overflowing.
- It is important to wait at least 24 hours after the set-up has been run before placing any living plants. This allows time to check that the heater and filter are working properly.
- Before the fish can be added the tank must be at the correct temperature, maturity and pH. Depending on which water company provides the water, it is either:
  - hard: a measure of the mineral salts dissolved in the water
  - soft: indicating fewer dissolved mineral salts
  - acid: pH up to 7
  - alkaline: pH from 7 up to 14
- Coldwater fish are adaptable to a wide range of pH but are most stable in water with a reading of pH between 7 and 8.5. Most tropical freshwater fish will live in water with a pH value between 6.5 and 7.5, which is about neutral in value, and from slightly soft to slightly hard water. There are kits available to check the pH levels.
- Once the tank is set up, it is best for it to be left for at least 3–4 weeks for the filtration system to mature; however, after 10 days the first few fish can be added, waiting a week to introduce the next few. The final number should be in place by 6 weeks, to give a healthy aquarium environment.
- Bacteria will develop in the filter sponge and assist in the breakdown of waste produced by the fish (ammonia is converted to nitrites by bacteria, nitrites are converted to nitrates in the filtration system). To ensure that both fish and live plants are healthy, maintenance of water quality must take place weekly.

A check on the nitrite level using a test kit will indicate whether a partial water change is required.

The nitrogen cycle in an aquarium

- Waste matter from the aquarium plants, uneaten food, faeces and urine from the fish will all contaminate the tank.
- As they decompose, ammonia is formed, which is poisonous to the fish.
- The bacteria in the water break down the ammonia into nitrites and then nitrates, which are harmless to fish and act as a fertiliser for the live plants in the tank. This completes the nitrogen cycle.

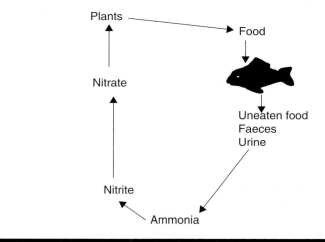

Feeding

Types of food:

- Live food (daphnia, brineshrimp and bloodworm)
- Commercial food (freeze-dried, tablet, dried flakes, floating food sticks and sinking granules)

The most convenient foods are the commercially produced flake or pellet foods. These provide the correct nutrient requirements and, unlike live foods, are free from the hazards of parasite or disease introduction.

Most coldwater fish kept in aquariums are omnivorous (feeding on insects and plant material). A good-quality flake food will provide the nutrients, vitamins and minerals required, but to keep the fish in good health, alternate this diet with other safe live food, such as daphnia or bloodworm.

Tropical freshwater fish also benefit from variety in their diet. Use of dried flake foods combined with frozen or live foods offered once or twice per week will maintain condition and health. If the fish are herbivorous, offer green foods, such as lettuce leaves, regularly .

Aquarium tank maintenance

Daily:

- Check the fish
- Check all the tank equipment
- Make sure that the temperature is correct
- Remove any uneaten food

Every two weeks:

- Test for pH and nitrite levels
- Do a partial water change
- Remove any dead plant material
- Remove any algal growth from the glass front and sides
- Suction off any debris seen on the sand or gravel substrate

Once a month:

- Clean the filter

Every 8–12 months:

- Replace fluorescent tube lights and air stones
- Service filter motor and air pump
- Take out and scrub all furniture and plastic plants to remove algae

Section 3
Nursing

Chapter 18
First Aid and Nursing

First aid

This is the emergency care and treatment of an animal with sudden illness or injury, before medical and surgical care (veterinary treatment) can be commenced. The main objectives at this time are to:

- Keep the animal alive
- Make it comfortable
- Assist in pain control
- Prevent its condition getting worse

Different situations require different approaches. Some situations will allow plenty of time to attend to injuries or problems and never be life threatening. Other situations are so severe the animal will die if urgent and skilled emergency care is not available.

First aid, being only the initial actions of someone attending or witnessing an accident, is very limited. It does not involve diagnosis or medical treatment of injuries, but is designed to preserve life and temporarily prevent a condition getting worse, if possible. It should allow time to get the animal to a veterinary surgeon who can diagnose the full extent of the condition, which is not always obvious at first.

Evaluating situations

Very severe

Must act immediately or the animal will die.

- The heart has stopped (*cardiopulmonary arrest*)
- Breathing is obstructed due to an object in the air passages
- Breathing has stopped
- Bleeding from a main artery or vein
- Acute allergic reaction to insect sting or other substance

Severe

Must act within one hour or the animal may die.

- Deep cuts and considerable blood loss
- Established shock
- Head injuries
- Breathing difficulties

Serious

Must act within 4–5 hours or more serious problems will develop that could be life threatening.

- Bone fractures that puncture through the skin (*compound fractures*)
- Spinal injuries
- Early stages of shock
- Difficulties in giving birth (*dystocia*)

Major

Must act within 24 hours to prevent further damage.

- Fractures with no skin injury (*simple fractures*)
- Prolonged vomiting and diarrhoea
- Foreign bodies in the eyes or ears

Initial management

(1) *Assess the situation and keep calm* – briefly examine the animal and note obvious injuries
(2) *Contact the veterinary practice* – for advice and to let them know you are coming
(3) *Ensure your own safety* – make sure the animal is properly restrained before handling and lifting, so that no one is bitten
(4) *Stop and cover any obvious bleeding* – use sterile dressings if possible, to prevent further contamination
(5) *Make sure the animal is able to breathe* – if the airway is obstructed, clear it
(6) *Treat for shock* – by maintaining the body temperature

Handling and transport

If the animal's life is in danger, then it must be moved. Injured animals are usually in pain, shocked and frightened and may attack anyone who tries to approach or handle them.

In order to protect both the handler and the animal from further harm or injury, great care is needed at this time.

- Slow, deliberate movements are essential
- A calm, soothing voice will help
- Handle the animal as little as possible
- Muzzle if necessary and only if the animal has no breathing difficulties
- Transport to the surgery

Before moving the animal, quickly assess the condition. This is referred to as *initial help* and if this can be started as soon as possible, the chances of survival are greatly improved. The initial assessment and help given must then be reported to the veterinary staff on arrival at the surgery, in order to reduce delay in treatment.

Checks to make are as follows:

- *Airway* – to ensure it is not obstructed; if it is, then clear it
- *Breathing* – to make sure this is possible and assist with artificial respiration if required
- *Heart and pulse* – check the beat, its rate and strength, and record the information. If the heart has stopped, then proceed with heart massage (see p. 229).

Species consideration is important when considering handling. The method for moving an injured dog will vary from the method used for horses, cattle or birds.

Small dogs, cats, rabbits and smaller pets

Transport in a pet carrier or in a cat-sized basket, making sure there are plenty of breathing holes. A lot of owners now own a cat cage, which is ideal for many species, provided there is plenty of space to stretch out (Fig. 18.1). Alternatively, and depending on the injury, the animal can be held in the owner's arms (Fig. 18.2).

Medium-sized dogs

If they only have minor injuries, then they may be encouraged to walk slowly. If they are not able to walk, then pick them up with one arm around the front of the forelegs and one around the hind legs (providing this is not contraindicated by the injuries), lift and hold against your body, with the legs hanging downward (Fig. 18.3).

Large breeds of dog or similar

These should only be lifted by more than one person, one supporting the head and chest and another supporting abdomen and hindquarters (Fig. 18.4). If the

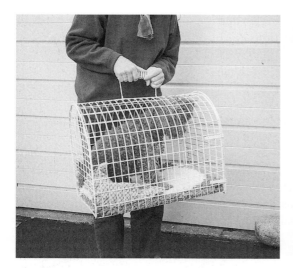

Fig. 18.1   Carrier cage for a small dog or cat.

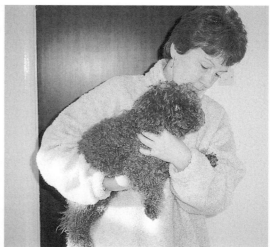

Fig. 18.2   Small dog held in arms.

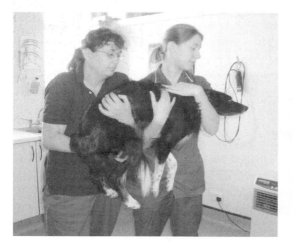

Fig. 18.3   Medium dog lift.

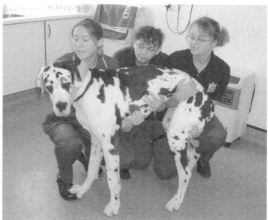

Fig. 18.4   Giant breed lift.

dog is too large for lifting, then with two or more handlers use a stretcher or blanket lift (Fig. 18.5). Pull the animal on to the blanket, lying on its side, and lift using the corners of the blanket or, if not enough handlers are available, simply drag the blanket, provided the surface is smooth. This blanket technique is also used for smaller animals with spinal injuries (Fig. 18.6).

Whatever the size of the injured animal, always lift in the correct manner; bend your knees before lifting rather than bending from the waist (Fig. 18.7). The handler's own back is less at risk, but if in doubt, get more help.

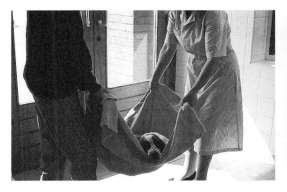

Fig. 18.5 Blanket lift requires two or more people for a large dog.

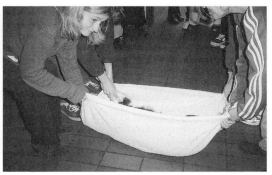

Fig. 18.6 Blanket lift for a smaller dog with spinal injuries.

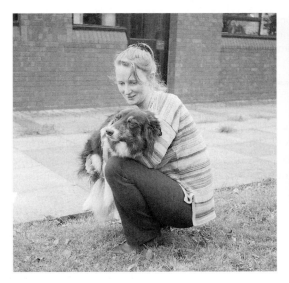

Fig. 18.7 Lift with straight back and bent knees to prevent back strain injury of the handler.

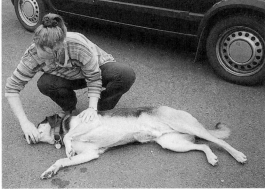

Fig. 18.8 Recovery position for an injured animal, keeping the airway straight.

Recovery position

As in human first aid, in animal first aid there is a *recovery position* in which to place the animal to ensure breathing is assisted and the heart is exposed for emergency procedures, if required (Fig. 18.8).

- Lie the animal on its right side
- Straighten head and neck
- The tongue is pulled forward and behind the canine tooth (to one side of the mouth)

- Remove any collar or harness
- Check the heart and pulse regularly

Other checks to make and record at this time include the following.

- Any signs of *bleeding* from the animal's surface or from a body opening, such as the mouth, rectum, vulva, prepuce or ears.
- *Colour* is checked by looking at the lining of the lower eyelid and the mucous membrane of the mouth and gums.

Colour of mucous membranes

- *Pale* – indicating shock or serious bleeding (internal or external)
- *Blue* – also referred to as *cyanotic*, indicates lack of oxygen to the tissue cells
- *Yellow* – also referred to as *jaundice*, can be caused by an excess of bile pigment in the bloodstream and usually involves the liver in some way
- *Red/congested* – indicates overoxygenation after exercise, in heat stroke cases or fever conditions

---

- The *capillary refill time* is checked. The upper lip is lifted and the gum over the top canine tooth is pressed. This squeezes the blood out of the surface capillaries, causing the area to go temporarily white. The refill time is the time it takes for the gum to become the normal pink colour again as the capillaries refill, usually $1–1\frac{1}{2}$ seconds. Any time longer than that is considered 'slow' and may indicate a degree of shock.
- *Rate and quality of the pulse*. This is taken in the groin area of the hind leg, on the femoral artery. This artery is exposed over the femur bone at this point, allowing the pulse to be taken. Another artery that may be used is the sublingual, under the animal's tongue, but this is only used in unconscious animals. *Rate* refers to the speed of the pulse, which is a reflection of the heart beat. The pulse should be taken for a full minute for a true recording. The *quality* of the pulse refers to whether it is strong, thready, weak or normal. In order to describe this, the handler must have some experience of pulse taking.
- *Breathing rate* is recorded, describing whether it is normal, slow, fast or shallow.
- *Body temperature* is taken if a thermometer is available. If not, then feel the extremities of the body, such as the feet and tail end. If the temperature is lower than it should be, the handler will feel this, because the normal body temperature of most animals (mammals and birds) is higher than that of humans.
- Record its *level of consciousness*; in other words, can the animal respond to stimuli like its name, a noise or sudden movement?

- Record any *unusual odour* on the animal's body, whether it comes from the animal's mouth, anus or coat.

Life-saving techniques

(1) The heart has stopped – *cardiac arrest*
(2) The breathing has stopped – *respiratory arrest*

The two above situations are jointly referred to as *cardiopulmonary arrest* (*pulmonary* refers to the vessels that take blood to the lungs and back to the heart).

The object of cardiopulmonary resuscitation is to restore heart and lung action and to prevent the irreversible brain damage that would happen if the tissues were deprived of oxygen for any length of time. Damage to body cells is thought to occur after 3–4 minutes following cardiac arrest. Therefore, being adequately prepared is the most important step in the management of these emergencies, and recognising that time is short if permanent damage to body tissues is to be avoided.

Cardiac compression (heart massage)

Small dogs or cats or other small animals

- Place in recovery position (on its right side, head and neck extended and tongue pulled forwards)
- Take hold of its chest between the thumb and fingers of the same hand, over the heart and just behind the elbows
- Support the body of the animal with the other hand on the lumbar spine area
- At all times, keep the head and neck in a straight line to assist breathing
- Squeeze the thumb and fingers of the hand over the heart together; this will compress the chest wall and the heart, which is squeezed between the ribs
- Repeat this action approximately 120 times per minute
- Watch for the heart contractions restarting

Medium-sized dogs and other species

- Place in the recovery position
- Put the heel of one hand on the top of the chest, just behind the elbow and over the heart (Figs 18.9, 18.10)
- Place the other hand either on top of the first hand or under the animal to support the heart as it is compressed
- Press down on to the chest with firm, sharp movements
- Repeat this action about 80–100 times per minute
- Watch for the heart contractions restarting

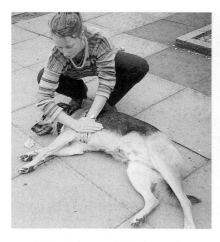

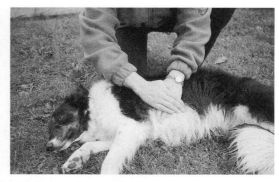

Fig. 18.10 Same hand position, behind the elbow, over the heart.

Fig. 18.9 Position for hands when doing cardiac massage.

Large, barrel-chested or fat dogs and other species

- Place on its back, with its head slightly lower than its body, if possible
- Put the heel of one hand on the abdominal end of the sternum (breast bone)
- Place the other hand on top of the first
- Press firmly on to the chest, pushing the hands forwards towards the head of the animal
- Press down in this way 80–100 times per minute
- Keep the head and neck straight during the procedure, at all times
- Watch for the heart restarting

With all animals, stop at 20-second intervals to check for heart beat or pulse, then continue.

Respiratory arrest

Whatever the cause, if the breathing has stopped, then it must urgently be restarted. Resuscitation methods do include the use of drugs that stimulate the heart and the breathing, but these are only administered by a veterinary surgeon and therefore are not a first aid procedure.

There are two methods for restarting the breathing:

(1) Artificial respiration – manual method
(2) Mouth-to-nose technique

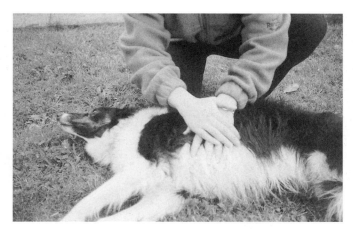

Fig. 18.11 For artificial respiration compression, hands are placed over the chest.

Artificial respiration

- Place in recovery position
- Clear airway of any blocking material
- Place a hand over the ribs, behind the shoulder bone (Fig. 18.11)
- Compress the chest with a sharp, downward movement
- Allow the chest to expand and then repeat the downward movement
- Repeat approximately every 3–5 seconds, until breathing restarts
- Keep head and neck straight at all times to maintain airway

Mouth-to-nose technique

- Place in recovery position
- Clear the airway
- Place a tissue or thin cloth over the animal's nose (for personal safety)
- Hold the animal's neck straight at all times
- Keep its mouth closed by holding upper and lower jaws together
- Breathe down its nose to inflate the lungs (Fig. 18.12)
- Repeat this inflation of the lungs at 3–5-second intervals
- Watch for the breathing restarting

This technique provides the animal with the unused oxygen in the handler's breath and their exhaled carbon dioxide, which helps to stimulate the breathing or gasp reflex in the animal.

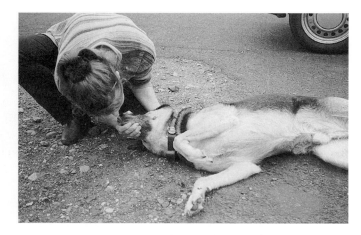

Fig. 18.12 Mouth-to-nose resuscitation with the airway kept straight and mouth held shut. The operator breathes down the nose.

Poisons

A poison or toxin is any substance which, on entry to the body in sufficient amounts, has a harmful effect on the individual. Poisons can gain entry to the body by various means:

- By mouth
- Via the lungs
- Absorbed through the skin surface
- Through a cut

Animals can be poisoned by a multitude of potentially toxic substances, many of which are ordinary household products. The source may be poisonous plants or toxic chemicals used or stored near the animal in the kitchen or utility room, where a dog or cat may have its bed. Such poisons would include:

- Pesticides for the garden, such as slug bait, herbicides, etc.
- Rodent killers, such as warfarin poison
- Paint and cleaning solutions for brushes
- Disinfectants such as bleach and toilet cleaners
- Drugs such as aspirin, blood pressure tablets and sleeping tablets

Very few poisons produce distinctive signs. Most cause non-specific signs, such as:

- Becoming aggressive, excited or depressed
- Unsteady on its feet

- Salivating, vomiting and/or having diarrhoea
- Abdominal pain and fitting-type episodes
- Pale, with lowered body temperature
- Slow capillary refill time

The owner knows best what is normal and what is unusual in their pet, so record all reported information and get in touch with the veterinary surgeon as soon as possible for advice on what to do next. If the owner knows the chemical involved and has the container or packet, take that to the veterinary surgeon too. Unless instructed to make the animal sick, do not attempt to do so as this may cause more harm.

Until the veterinary surgeon takes over:

- Place in recovery position
- Support for any breathing problems
- Keep warm to reduce shock
- Record pulse and heart rate
- Comfort and do not leave unattended

Get to the veterinary surgeon as quickly as possible.

Insect stings

These are usually more painful than harmful. However, it is possible that an animal may have an allergic reaction to the insect venom, or that the sting is near the airway and could obstruct breathing.

If the venom sac is imbedded in the skin, never squeeze it, as this may inject more venom into the animal. Remove carefully if possible, or leave it in place for the veterinary surgeon to remove in the safety of the practice.

Wasp stings are alkaline. Treatment is therefore with an acid solution, such as household vinegar in the form of a pad or compress.

Bee stings are acidic. Treatment is therefore with an alkali such as bicarbonate of soda mixed with water and soaked into a pad or compress.

Treatment aims to neutralise the situation. Unless someone has seen it bite, it is not always possible to know which insect is involved. If this is the case, then apply a cold compress or face flannel filled with ice cubes to the area to reduce the swelling and give some pain control.

Bleeding or haemorrhage

Bleeding or *haemorrhage* is the escape of blood from damaged blood vessels, and can cause serious problems. Bleeding heavily can decrease the circulating blood volume enough to cause shock. Bleeding that is less heavy may still cause the tissue cells to be deprived of oxygen, which could be permanently damaging. Even small losses of blood can delay wound healing and contribute to development of an infection. Therefore any loss potentially puts the animal at risk.

Bleeding is not always obvious; it may be *internal*, especially after a road traffic accident, so watch for the general signs:

- Colour is pale
- Attitude is dull or listless
- Appears thirsty
- The pulse and breathing rate are fast and may appear feeble
- Feet and tail are cold to the touch
- Body temperature is subnormal
- Capillary refill time is slow

If blood loss is severe, then signs include those of blood loss to vital organs, such as the following:

- The animal becomes restless and will not settle
- It has difficulty breathing
- It may have fitting-type episode
- The animal is unable to stand and becomes unconscious

For reporting purposes, the following information is useful to the veterinary surgeon:

- What type of blood vessel is damaged
- Where the injury is on the body
- When the bleeding started
- Whether the bleeding is internal or on the surface
- Treatments carried out so far

Which blood vessel is damaged?

- *Artery* – blood is bright red (oxygenated) in colour and comes out as spurts, which are synchronised with the heart beat
- *Vein* – blood is dark red (deoxygenated) in colour and is a steady flow
- *Capillary* – is bright red and seen as a steady ooze

Methods of arresting bleeding

The following methods are only for temporary application until the veterinary surgeon takes over.

Digital (finger) pressure

Used on a surface wound by pressing a sterile or clean pad of absorbent material on to the area to control the blood loss. Care must be used with this method in case there is a piece of metal, glass or wood imbedded in the wound tissues; pressing on this would push it deeper, where it would be harder to locate or may cause damage to internal structures.

This method can be used for about 5–15 minutes before tissues beyond must receive a reviving flow. Then pressure can be re-established.

Pressure points

In several locations around the body, major arteries are near the body surface. These tend to supply the extremities such as limbs and tail. Where they cross a bone, pressure can slow, or even stop, the supply reaching an area beyond. If the wound is on the extremity, these points can be used as a temporary measure.

- *Forelimbs* – the pressure is put on the inside or medial elbow area, to slow the brachial artery flow
- *Hind limbs* – the pressure is put on the same site used for pulse taking, in the groin area on the femur, to slow the femoral artery flow
- *Tail* – the pressure is applied to the ventral or underside of the base of the tail, to slow the coccygeal artery flow

These locations can be used for about 5–10 minutes, before allowing the blood to flow to restore distant tissues.

Pressure bandages

These may be used initially or after one or both of the above methods have been used to establish the extent of the injury.

Pressure bandages can only be applied to extremities, such as limbs and tail. They are applied tightly to constrict and slow the surface vessels supplying the area, thus limiting blood loss.

Plenty of padding material is applied over the dressing on the wound and is then tightly bandaged in place. If blood seeps through, then more padding is applied and bandaged in place.

This is still only a temporary measure to be used before arriving at the veterinary surgery, and will give about 1 hour of time before the tissues must be released from the tight bandage and flow restored.

Shock

Shock is a term used to describe a very complex and potentially fatal clinical syndrome which always involves insufficient blood to the tissues, resulting in lack of oxygen to the cells. Lack of oxygen to the cells is called *tissue hypoxia* and this can be fatal if not corrected.

When blood is lost from the body, the body tries to compensate by redistributing blood to vital structures like the brain and heart, at the expense of other organs like kidneys, skin, intestines and muscles. Organs can be severely damaged by the resulting tissue hypoxia.

The causes of shock vary, but some examples are:

- Blood loss from damaged vessels
- Trauma injuries to tissues from a road traffic accident
- Pain due to injury or surgical procedures
- Heart problems that interfere with its normal pumping action
- Infections that cause blood to 'pool out' in the capillary beds, by affecting the walls of the blood vessels

The *signs of shock* include:

- Pale colour (Fig. 18.13)
- Cold extremities
- Weak, or slipping into an unconscious state
- Increase in the heart rate and breathing
- Slow capillary refill time of longer than two seconds (Fig. 18.14)

Until the animal can be treated by a veterinary surgeon, the handler must start the preventive shock procedure. Maintaining body temperature is probably the

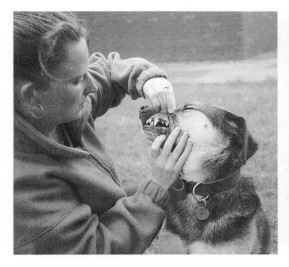

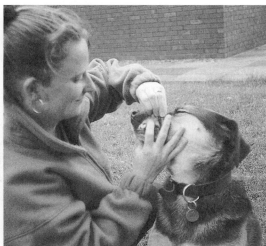

Fig. 18.13   Mucous membrane colour check.   **Fig. 18.14**   Capillary refill time check.

single most useful thing that can be done. If the body is not allowed to shut down the peripheral vessels to the limbs and tail, shock will be at least delayed and possibly even prevented.

Shock takes three forms:

(1) *Impending* – it is expected to happen, bearing in mind the events or injuries
(2) *Established* – it is in place and the animal must have urgent medical treatment involving whole-blood transfusions or use of plasma expanders
(3) *Irreversible* – treatment is unlikely to save the animal's life as systems are too damaged

Treatment is aimed at not allowing shock to move beyond the impending stage. To achieve this:

* Maintain body temperature by wrapping in blankets or towels (Fig. 18.15) and keep massaging or rubbing the extremities to stimulate the blood flow. Never use artificial heat as the temperature may get too high
* Position the head slightly lower than the body to encourage the blood flow to the brain
* Stop any further blood loss
* Assist the animal to breathe by placing in the recovery position, and give artificial respiration if breathing stops
* Record the pulse
* Get to the veterinary surgery as quickly as possible

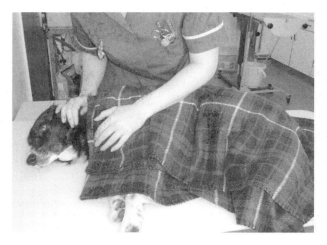

Fig. 18.15 Maintaining body temperature.

Hyperthermia (heat stroke)

Heat stroke results from an excessive rise in body temperature caused by high environmental temperatures. Dogs and cats do not lose body temperature through the skin due to their dense coats and lack of sweat glands. Therefore to eliminate excess body heat they use the respiratory system, inhaling cool air through the nose and exhaling hot air from the body through the mouth. The faster this exchange occurs, the faster their body will cool down, which is why dogs pant after exercise.

Heat stroke is rarely seen in cats, and in dogs it usually occurs because the animal has been confined, on a hot day, with no access to shade, or in a car/vehicle with insufficient ventilation.

N.B. On a hot day the temperature in a car soon becomes higher than the environmental temperature, even if windows are left open.

When the environmental temperature exceeds the animal's body temperature, it ultimately becomes impossible to maintain body temperature within normal limits for that animal.

Heat stroke affects all dogs, but those most at risk, if exposed to excess heat, are:

- Those with thick dense coats
- Overweight animals
- Short-nosed breeds
- Animals with heart conditions
- Elderly animals
- Animals with medical conditions that affect the breathing

Panting becomes ineffective and the body temperature will rise rapidly, death follows quickly if the body temperature is not immediately reduced.

Signs of heat stroke include:

- Excess panting and salivation
- Bright red mucous membranes (check the gums)
- Vomiting
- Excitement/anxiety
- Disoriented
- Collapsed/unable to stand
- Body temperature high (41–43°C)

It is essential to reduce body temperature urgently:

(1) Remove the animal from the hot environment
(2) Cool using:
    - a pack of frozen vegetables held on the neck area

- wrap in towel/blanket soaked with cold water, and continue to hose water over the soaked wrapping, keeping clear of the face
(3) Monitor the animal's body temperature
(4) If collapsed, put into the recovery position to assist breathing
(5) If conscious, encourage to drink restricted amounts of water continuously (if unrestricted, the animal may swallow too much too quickly and cause vomiting)
(6) Treat for shock if the temperature falls below normal

Hypothermia

Hypothermia is commonly seen in young or small animals, due to an inability to control body temperature within normal limits. This may be caused by illness or accident, leaving the animal unable to restore temperature loss unless assisted.

Signs:

- The animal appears sleepy or lethargic
- Its movement becomes weaker
- It is unconscious

Treatment:

- If the animal is wet, dry it by rubbing vigorously with a towel
- Wrap, using a lightweight covering, to preserve heat
- Increase the environmental temperature but do not overheat
- Monitor constantly by taking temperature and do not leave unattended

Bone fractures

A fracture refers to a crack in the surface of a bone or a complete break in a bone structure. The objectives of first aid for fractures are to prevent the situation getting worse and make the animal comfortable for transportation to the veterinary surgery.

The causes of bone fracture are varied and include:

- Road traffic accidents
- The animal landing badly after jumping
- Muscles contracting to break small bones, particularly in the legs of racing dogs or horses
- Bone disease that has weakened the bone structure

Types of fracture

- *Simple* – the bone is broken but there is no connecting skin injury (Fig. 18.16)
- *Compound* – the bone is broken and there is a wound connecting to the skin, or the bone is protruding through the skin. A badly handled simple fracture can become a compound fracture

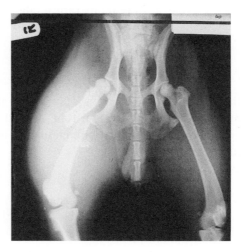

Fig. 18.16   X-ray shows fractured right femur and extent of tissue swelling.

The signs indicating a fracture include:

- Loss of use of the affected limb, will not bear weight
- Pain on handling or will not allow handling
- Unusual position or shape to the limb
- Swelling and bruising
- Unusual movement of the limb

The best treatment for fractured bones is to get the animal to the veterinary surgery quickly, but taking care to cause no further injuries by careless handling. Some fractures are also complicated by damage to surrounding tissues, such as blood vessels, nerves or organs.

Depending on the fracture, first aid aims to:

- Stop any bleeding.
- Clean and cover any wounds.
- Immobilise the fracture site. This is only possible if the joints above and below the site can be immobilised by a splint. If splinting is possible, always apply

the splint to the limb in the position in which it is found. For example, if the foot and carpals of the foreleg are now positioned sideways instead of facing front, do not correct the position – splint it.

Materials that can be used for splinting include:

- Rolled-up magazine or newspaper
- A ruler or piece of wood
- Cardboard
- A matchstick

If a splint is not possible then:

- Confine on plenty of bedding
- Comfort and do not leave unattended
- Treat for shock
- Get to the veterinary surgery

What can be splinted?

- *Forelimb* – from elbow to toes (*phalanges*)
- *Hind limb* – from stifle to toes
- *Tail*

Wounds

A wound is damage to the continuous structure of any tissue in the body.

Healing of a wound

First-intention healing

Takes place in wounds that:

- Are not contaminated with grit, soil or micro-organisms
- Have clean-cut edges that can be held together
- Have been cleaned within one hour of injury

In this type of healing, the edges rejoin by ten days after injury.

Second-intention healing or granulation

Takes place in wounds that:

- Are contaminated with grit, soil and micro-organisms
- Have jagged edges and possibly sections of skin missing
- Have not been cleaned within two hours of injury
- Have edges that gape open
- Become infected

This type of healing can take weeks to months.

Types of wound

Wounds are described as being open or closed. The *closed* wound is one that does not penetrate the whole thickness of the skin as a structure, such as bruises or blood blisters (*haematoma*), or pockets of blood from a small damaged blood vessel. Treatment of these injuries involves use of a cold compress, such as ice cubes held in a face flannel, immediately after injury, to reduce the swelling of local tissues and help control pain. This treatment is only useful immediately after injury.

Open wounds are those with damage to surface tissue and some bleeding. They are named according to the manner of the damage, and whether or not tissue is missing:

- *Incised* – these have clean-cut edges, are painful due to surface nerve ending damage and tend to bleed freely. Caused by sharp-edged materials such as glass, metal or knife blade.
- *Lacerated* – these have very jagged flaps of skin and sometimes skin sections are missing (*avulsed*). However, because tissue is torn and stretched, they are less painful than incised wounds and do not bleed much. Caused by bite injuries, barbed wire or road traffic accident.
- *Puncture* – these wounds have a long, narrow track deep into the tissues, with only a small skin entry scab over the track. The scab holds any microbes in the track. The wound is caused by sharp, pointed objects, such as teeth in bite wounds, nails and thorns. These will all be contaminated with microbes, which are then left in the damage track to multiply, causing a local infection to develop. This local infection is held in the track area and, as it increases in size, is called an *abscess*. These are very painful, often causing loss of limb function.
- *Abrasions* – these have torn, ragged skin edges, with many contaminants embedded in the damaged areas. They are caused by a glancing blow or by being dragged along the ground briefly in a road traffic accident. The tissues tend to be torn and the damage only in the surface layers of the skin, so there is not much bleeding.

Wound care

The sooner an open wound is cleaned using a water-based antiseptic solution, the more chance there is that infection will not develop. Solutions used for wound cleaning must not cause any further inflammation or damage to the wound, and therefore should not contain any detergent.

If micro-organisms in the wound are prevented from multiplying, it could mean the difference between the wound healing within ten days (*first intention*) and the delayed healing of the second-intention or granulation method.

Solutions to use:

- Tap water
- 0.9% sodium chloride from a drip bag

Once cleaned, always cover the wound to prevent contamination and further aggravation of the area by the animal.

Eye injuries

Any animal with eye injuries will be sight impaired and in pain. It is very important to approach slowly and talk to the animal so that it is warned of your approach. The animal will be frightened and could injure the handler unless precautions are observed and correct handling techniques used (Fig. 18.17).

The types of injury seen include the following.

Chemicals

These can cause serious injury to the eye structures. Always irrigate as soon as possible, using tap water to remove any chemical. Do not leave unattended and seek medical help.

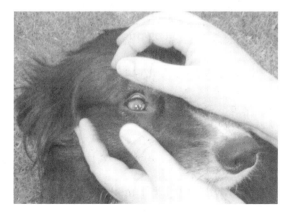

Fig. 18.17   Examine the eye carefully, touching the lids only.

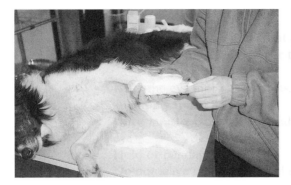

Fig. 19.1 The area to be bandaged is protected with a padding material, between the toes and dew claw.

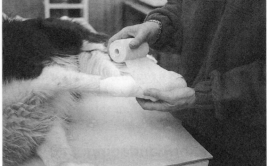

Fig. 19.2 A protective layer covers the bandage.

Aims of bandaging

- It must be comfortable. If applied too tightly, the animal will try to remove the bandage or the surface tissues will be damaged by the animal's constant licking.
- Prevents the animal interfering with the area under the bandage.
- Limits movement in the case of broken bones or tissue damage and therefore limits pain.
- Stays on for the required amount of time.
- Looks neat but will do the job until professional help is reached.

Watch out for:

- Smells coming from the bandage
- Discomfort
- Interference or self-mutilation to try and remove the bandage
- Overexercising
- Bandage getting wet or dirty
- Any signs of ill health

If any of the above are seen in an animal with a bandage, report to the veterinary surgeon straight away for advice.

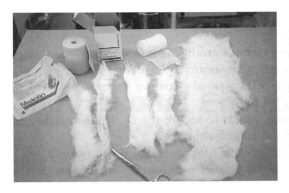

Fig. 19.3 Prepare all materials prior to restraint of the animal.

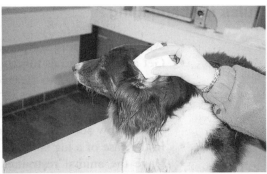

Fig. 19.4 Ear bandage. First protect the wound with a dressing.

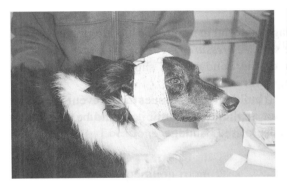

Fig. 19.5 Hold dressing in place with injured ear flap bandaged against the top of the head.

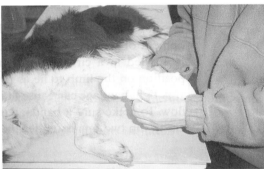

Fig. 19.6 The padding.

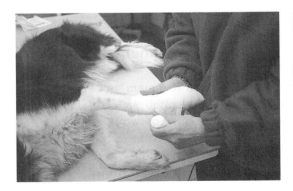

Fig. 19.7 The bandage.

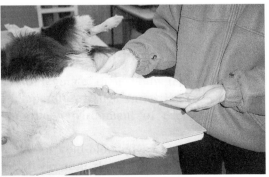

Fig. 19.8 The top protective layer.

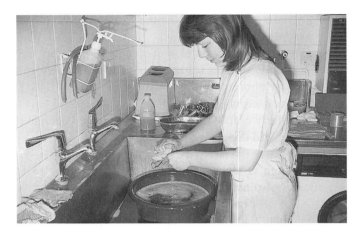

Fig. 20.6   Instruments in cold water/detergent ready for cleaning.

There is a mixture of personnel in this area:

- Those that are scrubbed up and part of the operating team and who may only touch the sterile operating site.
- Those of the non-sterile team who have various duties to perform but are not involved with the surgical areas. They will operate the monitoring systems, maintain anaesthetics and other equipment which supports the surgical procedure.

Personal hygiene for the non-scrubbed team is important although not to the same high standard as the operating team. Non-scrubbed staff have the jobs of:

- Producing equipment required, at the appropriate time
- Tidying away equipment
- Preparing for the next operation

There should be minimal traffic through the theatre because movement increases the distribution of micro-organisms in the atmosphere and therefore could increase the incidence of wound infections. There should be a ventilation system which replaces theatre air with clean air approximately ten times per hour in order to prevent airborne contamination.

On completion of the day's surgical procedures:

- Collect used instruments, place in cold water/detergent solutions ready for cleaning (Fig. 20.6)
- Collect and dispose of all waste
- Spot check and clean all surfaces with disinfectant
- Restock disposable equipment

- Check all other supplies and equipment
- Wipe down walls, operating table and doors with disinfectant
- Vacuum floor for any hair/coat material
- Mop the floor, starting farthest from the exit door and working towards it
- Ventilate room
- Before next operation, 'wet dust' all surfaces with antiseptic solution

---

Hygiene terms

- *Sterilisation* – the removal or destruction of all living micro-organisms including bacterial spores.
- *Disinfectants* – will kill pathogenic micro-organisms.
- *Antiseptics* – prevent micro-organism from multiplying and therefore infection fails to develop.
- *Asepsis* – is a state of being free from micro-organisms.

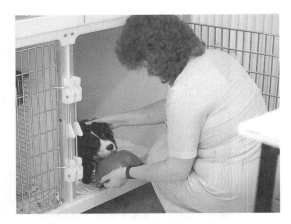

Fig. 21.4   Postoperatively patients will need to be encouraged to feed.

Feeding may also be contraindicated for a number of reasons:

- Scheduled for surgery and must have an empty stomach
- Medical condition
- After surgery to the gastrointestinal tract
- Requires blood tests
- Is vomiting and/or has diarrhoea

Hygiene

Regular checks are made through the day to make sure no animal lies in a body discharge (Fig. 21.5). After moving the animal from a soiled housing or kennel, check to see if samples need to be collected for investigations.

Mark the cage details, with collection times, then clean and disinfect. To prevent animals from getting soiled, grills may be covered with a layer of bedding to allow a soak-away effect for use with incontinence pads.

Temperature control

Pre- and postoperative patients need assistance to regain lost body heat and prevent the establishing of shock. Heat can be provided by:

- Environmental thermostat controls
- Kennels with underfloor heating
- Heated underpads (Fig. 21.6)
- Incubator for small or newborn animals

It is important never to overheat but simply to support body temperature. Use of heat lamps can be harmful if the animal is unable to move away; it could

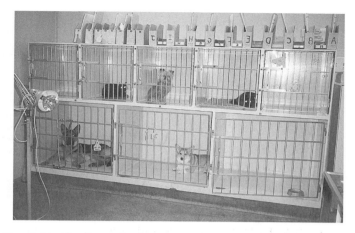

Fig. 21.5   Hospital holding kennels allow easy monitoring for signs of soiling.

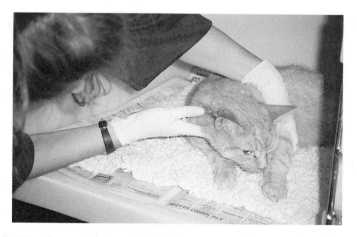

Fig. 21.6   Bedding for warmth postoperatively will support body temperature.

overheat and even suffer skin burns if the lamp is too close. Always keep the lamp a minimum of one metre from the body of the animal to avoid any over-heating or burns.

Recumbent patients

- Use deep bedding to prevent pressure on any bony areas (Fig. 21.7)
- Do not allow to remain in soiled kennel
- Use incontinence pads
- Assist drinking to prevent dehydration
- Assist eating, giving small meals often
- Groom and clean away any food on the coat after feeding

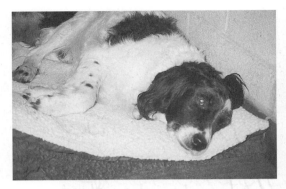

Fig. 21.7 Plenty of bedding for recumbent patients.

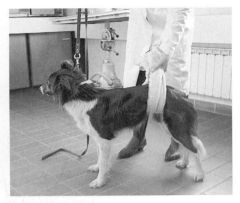

Fig. 21.8 Assist to stand using sling to support hindquarters.

- Unless contraindicated, encourage limb movements to stimulate circulation (Fig. 21.8)
- Turn the animal every 1–2 hours to prevent fluid pooling in the chest due to shallow breathing
- Rub and stroke body to stimulate surface circulation, generating heat and fluid movement within the tissues
- Spend time playing with the animal
- Assist to urinate or check indwelling urinary catheter

Handling

Use coat care and grooming as an excuse to handle. Also wipe any discharges from nose, eye or ears and keep the area around the mouth moistened using damp cotton wool to simulate the animal's own grooming routines. This will all contribute to a feeling of well-being for the animal, accustoms them to the nursing staff and promotes recovery.

Isolation and barrier nursing

If the patient has a suspected contagious or zoonotic disease, it must be moved to the isolation area. Barrier nursing follows strict rules to prevent crossinfection between routine patients or staff members. Barrier nursing involves:

- Protective clothing – disposable apron, intact gloves and mask if necessary
- Change of footwear
- Required drugs and medical equipment for patient care

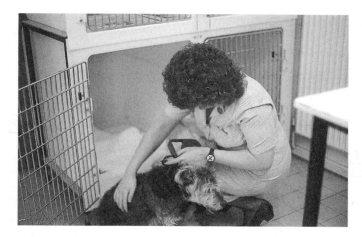

Fig. 21.9   TLC to promote recovery.

- Cleaning equipment for unit use only
- Feeding materials and cleaning of bowls in the unit
- One member of staff to work in isolation only and not handle any other patients

Medication

For any patient in the hospital, always check:

- Timings
- Dosage per day
- Whether tablet or injection required and/or assistance
- Route

Fluid therapy

This will involve:

- Care and maintenance of intravenous catheters
- Preventing patient interference (use of Elizabethan collar)
- Checking the fluid is running in properly
- Monitoring quantities delivered
- Changing drip fluid bags on instruction
- Monitoring hydration status
- Recording and reporting all details

Environmental enrichment

- Preferred foods
- Assisting to eat and drink; expect this to be time consuming but time well spent
- Comfort in the cage, kennel or housing
- Enough space
- Music helps calm both humans and animals
- Do not mix species
- Toys are helpful for long-stay patients, providing interest and, if not contraindicated, activity too
- TLC (Fig. 21.9)

Chapter 22
Monitoring Temperature, Pulse and Respiration

The skill of observation and monitoring life signs is essential to nursing of any species of animal. It involves the comparing of normal behaviour against that which is abnormal. Time spent with an animal, using all senses, is most important. The nurse should be capable of recognising minute changes to the animal's life signs and temperament.

Temperature, pulse and respiration or breathing all vary in animals due to environmental temperature, recent exercise, stress situations and excitement. Increase or decrease in the rate of these life signs can also indicate a problem with a body system or that a disease is present. These life signs should be checked hourly or, until an animal is stabilised, more frequently.

Temperature

Most species can regulate their body temperature in response to internal and external influences to within a very narrow range, due to homeostasis. Taking the body temperature of cold-blooded species like reptiles is not useful because they rely on environmental sources for their own heat. The ability of warm-blooded animals to control their own body temperature may disappear when ill or injured.

Heat loss methods

- Sweating
- Panting
- Drinking water
- Position – spread out, seeking a cold surface to lie on
- Vasodilation – surface blood vessels increase in size to lose body heat

Heat gain methods

- Shivering
- Position – curled up
- Vasoconstriction – surface blood vessels reduce in size to reduce body heat loss

Table 22.1   Normal temperatures.

Species	Celsius	Fahrenheit
Dog	38.3–38.7	100.9–101.7
Cat	38.0–38.5	100.4–101.6
Guinea pig	38.4–40	102.2–104
Rabbit	38.5–40	101.5–104
Rat	37.5	99.9
Hamster	36–38	98–101
Mouse	37.5	99.5

Differences between:

Clinical thermometer

Contains mercury
Triangular in shape
Scale difference
Constriction near bulb
Needs to be shaken down before use
Short shaft

Laboratory thermometer

Contains spirit or mercury
Circular in shape
Scale difference
No constriction
Needs no shaking down before use
Long shaft

Temperature increase may be seen:

- In infections and fevers
- After recent exercise
- In fear or excitement
- In heat stroke (*hyperthermia*)
- In hot weather

Temperature decrease may be seen:

- In shock and severe bleeding
- In exposure cases (*hypothermia*)
- In hibernation
- In anaesthesia
- Before impending death (moribund animal)
- Immediately before *parturition* (giving birth)

Pulse

The pulse is used as a means of checking the heart (*cardio*) and blood (*vascular*) function. With each heart beat, the artery walls expand and contract in size to allow the created wave of blood to pass and maintain its speed of flow. This is called the pulse. If there is a change in the heart function or the volume of blood then there will be a reflected change in the pulse rate (speed) or character.

Words used to describe the pulse include:

- Intermittent
- Thready – slow, soft pulse
- Irregular
- Strong
- Weak

A normal pulse is usually described as regular, strong or firm. It is essential that time is spent feeling pulses, both normal and abnormal, to increase the operator's ability to assess the state of the animal. This will also dramatically decrease the time it takes to find the animal's pulse.

The pulse is taken where an artery runs close to the body surface. Each pulsation corresponds with the contraction of the right and left ventricles of the heart.

Sites used

- Femoral artery located in the groin region on the medial aspect of the femur of the hind leg.
- Digital artery located on the cranial or anterior surface of the hock region of the hind leg.
- Coccygeal artery located on the ventral (underside) aspect of the base of the tail just above the rectum.
- Lingual artery located on the ventral (underside) aspect of the tongue. However, this site can only be used in unconscious or anaesthetised animals.

The most common site used to take the pulse is the femoral artery on the hind leg. Before taking the pulse, the animal must be suitably restrained so two people make the task much easier.

Taking the pulse

- Get the animal used to being restrained.
- Once the animal is settled, take the pulse by placing the fingers over the chosen artery.
- When properly located, using a watch with a second hand, count the pulse for one minute. Never shorten this period because the pulse can change quickly and a reading of less than one minute could be inaccurate and therefore useless.
- Write down the pulse count at the end of the minute.
- Relax the restraint of the animal and praise.

Table 22.2 Normal pulse recording.

Species	Pulse rate (beats per minute)
Dog	60–180*
Cat	110–180
Rabbit	150–300
Guinea pig	230–320
Hamster	300–600
Mouse	500–600

*The pulse range in dogs is due to the size variation from toy breeds (nearer the 180 end of the range) to giant breeds (nearer the 60 end of the range).

Pulse terms

Dysrhythmia – indicates that the pulse and heart rate are not synchronised. The pulse is lower due to the heart pumping blood inefficiently.
Sinus arrhythmia – refers to the pulse rate increase on breathing in and decrease on breathing out. This is often considered to be normal.
Fast pulse – occurs when the tissues are not getting enough oxygen and the heart is compensating by speeding up to meet the body's needs. Fast pulse can be normal after exercise.

Pulse increase

- Exercise
- Excitement or stress
- Heart/valve disease
- Shock or loss of blood
- Pain
- High temperature/fever

Pulse decrease

- Sleep
- Unconsciousness
- Heart disease
- Other disease condition

Table 22.3 Normal respiration rates.

Species	Rate (breaths per minute)
Dog	10–30
Cat	20–30
Rabbit	35–65
Guinea pig	110–150
Hamster	75
Gerbil	90–140
Mouse	100–250

Respiration

Normal breathing is almost silent, although air flow may be heard in the airways. The breathing and cardiovascular systems are very closely linked so a change in one is mirrored in the other. If the blood gas levels of oxygen or carbon dioxide become abnormal this will be seen in the animal's colour, its pulse rate and character and in the breathing.

Certain breeds of dog and cat may, because of airway anatomy (short-nosed breeds), make considerable breathing sounds and this is normal.

There should be a rhythm to the breathing, in that the time between breathing in and out should be equal. The breathing can be varied by use of the voluntary or skeletal muscles of the chest or thorax.

The ability to voluntarily alter breathing means that the rate can only be taken once the animal has settled. Any obvious restraint will probably cause the breathing to increase in response. The reading is taken on either breathing in or breathing out and when the animal:

- Is not panting
- Has not recently exercised
- Has not been stressed by overrestraint
- Is not asleep

The respiratory rate is taken when the animal is calm, awake and comfortable. After close observation by the operator, a decision is taken to count on breathing in or breathing out. The recording is timed using a watch with a second hand for one minute. Note is also made of the depth of breathing.

Causes of respiration increase

- Shock or haemorrhage
- Recent exercise
- Pain
- Excitement or fear

- Heat stroke
- Medical disease, especially of the respiratory system

Causes of respiration decrease

- Unconsciousness
- Sleep
- Poisons
- Low body temperature (hypothermia)

Breathing terms

- *Tachypnoea* – rapid, shallow breathing.
- *Hyperpnoea* – panting.
- *Apnoea* – no breathing taking place.
- *Cheyne–Stokes* – irregular breathing (deep breaths, then fast shallow breaths) seen shortly before death.
- *Dyspnoea* – difficulty breathing in or out and often painful.

Signs of difficult breathing

- Forced breathing out
- Flaring of nostrils
- Extended head and neck
- Elbows rotated away from the chest
- Breathing through the mouth
- Exaggerated movements of the chest and abdomen
- Sounds
- Unable to settle

Chapter 23
Pharmacy and the Administration of Drugs

Pharmacology is the science of drugs:

- The way in which the drug affects the body
- Its absorption into the body
- Its metabolism by the body
- The method used by the body to finally excrete it

Dispensing is the giving out of drugs to the owner of the animal requiring them, either by the veterinary practice at which the owner is registered or by taking a prescription to a dispensing chemist.

Drugs are administered in various ways. This is often dependent on the drug target in the body, how quickly the effect of the drug is required and the ability of the owner to give the drug.

Routes

Oral (Fig. 23.1)

This is the most frequently used route for drugs because the owner can treat at home. The products are supplied in various forms, from tablet to powder. Many tablets have an outer coating and therefore should never be broken up or crushed in case the action of the drug is reduced. Reasons for coating tablets include:

- Protection of the drug from moisture
- To hide an unpleasant taste
- To assist in identification
- To protect the drug from the hydrochloric acid in the stomach (enteric coated)
- Protection of the stomach from the irritant effect of a drug

Oral administration can have disadvantages.

- If the animal is vomiting
- Absorption can be slow and some of the drug may not be absorbed at all
- The presence of food may reduce the drug's effect
- The animal may refuse to swallow the drug
- Owner is unable to give the drug to the animal

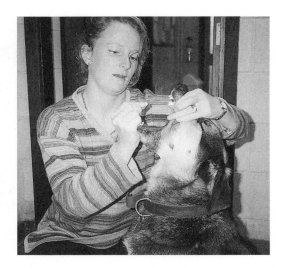

Fig. 23.1 The mouth is opened wide so that the tablet can then be placed at the back of the throat for swallowing.

Parenteral

A route other than by mouth. It usually refers to or is taken to mean 'by injection'. Any drug administered by this method must be sterile and the method involves some skin site cleaning and personal hygiene. The most frequently used injection methods are:

- *Subcutaneous* – into the connective tissues below the skin (below the hypodermis). This method is for non-irritant drugs and absorption is slow.
- *Intramuscular* – directly into a muscle body (hind leg or back). This method is used for small volumes of drug only and can be painful but the drug is more rapidly absorbed than by the subcutaneous route.
- *Intravenous* – into a surface vein (foreleg, hind leg or neck vein). This method places the drug directly into the bloodstream and has very rapid action.

Other injection routes less frequently used are:

- *Epidural* – into the vertebral canal to give spinal pain control (*analgesia*)
- *Intra-articular* – directly into a joint
- *Intradermal* – into the skin structure

Topical

These drug preparations are applied to a surface tissue like the skin, eyes or ears (Fig. 23.2). They are absorbed into either just the surface of the skin or mucous membranes or the structure of the skin, depending on the material used to carry the drug. Some topical drugs may be able to move into body systems which is

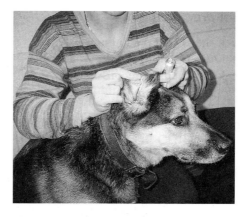

Fig. 23.2   The ointment/cream is applied to the affected area on the ear flap.

why the operator must immediately wash off any drug that contacts their skin. Types of carriers used include:

- Water to place wettable powder against the skin
- Petroleum jelly as ointment that melts with body heat
- Oil and water together as a cream, which will penetrate into the skin layers
- Detergent-based products as medicated shampoos to cover the skin surface before rinsing off

Pharmacology and dispensing

For safe drug administration, be sure that the following are checked and confirmed before medication is given.

Is it the right:

- drug?
- patient?
- dose?
- route for the drug?
- time interval?

Administer the right drug

- Check label
- Check against the animal's medical record, if available
- If the writing is illegible on the medical record, get it clarified
- Understand the difference between trade names and generic names

practices, saddlers and animal wholesale outlets such as animal feed and farm merchants.

(3)   P – these are pharmacy medicines supplied by veterinary practices and dispensing chemist chains.

(4)   GSL – these are general sales list medicines and can be supplied and sold by pet shops and other outlets.

The group symbol is found on the drug container label and any outer packaging.

A special category of drugs, those that could be abused by humans, are known as the *controlled drugs* (CD). The legislation applicable here is the Misuse of Drugs Regulations 1985, which is divided into five schedules. These schedules are set out in decreasing order of the need to control.

- *Schedule 1* – includes drugs like cannabis and hallucinogenic drugs such as LSD, which are considered non-therapeutic and are therefore not legally held in veterinary practice for the purpose of treating animals.
- *Schedule 2* – includes the opiate analgesics (pain control) like morphine pethidine, and etorphine (anaesthetic agent). These drugs are POM and records are kept on their ordering, supply, safe storage and, if out of date or not required, their destruction.
- *Schedule 3* – includes barbiturates (used for anaesthesia, control of epilepsy and euthanasia), some minor stimulant drugs and some analgesics (pain control). These drugs are POM and must have safe storage and purchase records.
- *Schedule 4* – includes the benzodiazepine drugs such as valium and diazepam (used to reduce stress). When these drugs are given to patients within the veterinary practice (for example, in injectable form only) they are exempt from restrictions.
- *Schedule 5* – contains preparations with only traces of otherwise controlled drugs, such as cocaine, codeine (cough mixture) and morphine (kaolin and morphine for diarrhoea treatment). The levels of drug are so small that they are exempt from restrictions.

Some drugs carry special risks. Harmful products may produce an acute effect immediately after contact whereas others may accumulate over time and constant exposure will be necessary before their effect on the operator or nurse is seen.

High-risk products include:

- Certain hormone products, like those used to postpone oestrus
- Cytotoxic drugs – those used in the treatment of cancers
- Gaseous anaesthetic agents like halothane
- Certain antibiotics
- Antifungal powders – those used to treat ringworm
- Insecticides

Drugs glossary

Group	Definition
Anabolic	Promotes growth of body tissue
Analgesic	Relieves or prevents pain
Anthelmintic	Kills internal parasitic worms
Antibiotic	Disrupts or destroys bacteria
Anticoagulant	Prevents blood from clotting
Antidiuretic	Hormone which reduces urine output
Corticosteroids	Suppress inflammation
Diuretic	Increases urine production
Emetic	Causes vomiting
Sedative	Reduces awareness of surroundings
Vaccine	Stimulates the production of antibodies

Chapter 24
Isolation and Quarantine

Isolation

Isolation is required when an animal is believed to have, or has, a disease that can be passed on to others (*contagious*). There is also protective isolation for susceptible animals, e.g. unvaccinated puppies and kittens. In their case, the isolation is in the owner's home and garden, which becomes the controlled environment.

In many veterinary practices and hospitals there is a purpose-built isolation unit where contagious animals can be housed and nursed. In other types of group housing, this type of facility may have to be created, as the need arises. Home-made isolation may involve use of a foldaway cage or cage box in a non-animal area of the unit which can be carefully controlled.

Infectious diseases of the dog and cat needing isolation

Dog	Cat
Distemper	Feline infectious peritonitis
Hepatitis	Feline leukaemia virus
Leptospirosis	Feline panleucopenia
Kennel cough	Cat flu
Ringworm	Ringworm
Sarcoptic mange	

The affected animal is housed in such a manner as to prevent other animals coming into contact with the disease-producing organisms it will be shedding. Micro-organisms can be shed via:

- Urine
- Faeces
- Blood
- Discharges from eyes, ears, nose, mouth, prepuce, vulva or a wound
- Respiratory tract via sneezing or coughing
- Vomit

Bearing in mind the exit routes for contagious diseases, isolation must follow disease management rules:

- One member of staff specifically allocated to the isolation area
- Change into protective clothing
- Change into protective footwear or set up a footbath containing disinfectant
- Additional protection of gloves and mask
- The unit must contain all required food preparation equipment and food bowls
- Cleaning equipment to be used in the unit should be kept there
- Instruments used here are cleaned here
- Safe disposal of soiled bedding, faeces, urine, vomit, blood and saliva, which may contain infectious micro-organisms
- Medical supplies to be available in the unit

An isolation facility must have an area for kennels, cages and a run area, for housing of various species, with a good ventilation system. Any treatments must take place within this area, which requires a sink unit, examination table and basic medical supplies. All cleaning equipment and feeding supplies for patients must be for use in isolation only. Hygiene is essential to assist the full recovery of the patient. Thorough cleaning of all surfaces, feeding equipment and bedding materials will reduce the number of micro-organisms present.

All staff members must disinfect or change footwear and overalls and wash hands in antiseptic solution before leaving to move through the other areas of the animal housing. It is essential never to put healthy animals or humans at risk by careless behaviour. There is also the possibility that the disease may transmit from animals to human carers (known as a *zoonone* or *zoonotic disease*).

Quarantine

This refers to the detention of animals coming into the UK for a set period of time, in isolation from other animals, in order to screen for disease (Fig. 24.1). Under the Rabies Order 1974 (as amended) any animal landed in the UK without a licence or PET passport may be directed to quarantine, exported or destroyed, and its owner prosecuted.

Quarantine time will vary depending on the species involved. For dogs and cats, the time is six calendar months to be spent in a quarantine kennel, in order to screen for rabies in particular. For other species, the times and locations vary, but will involve separation from the main group of animals or birds at a given location. In this manner, the resident animals are not put at risk by the newcomer.

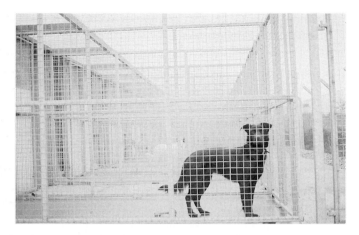

Fig. 24.1   The dog is kept isolated from others in its own housing and run area.

Quarantine of dogs and cats in the UK

In March 1999 the government proposed changes to the quarantine laws, as recommended by the Kennedy Advisory Group. The Kennedy Advisory Group was appointed to look at the existing regulations and make recommendations for replacing quarantine.

The new scheme proposed to allow dogs and cats coming from EU countries, certain other European countries and rabies-free islands to enter the UK without having to undergo quarantine, provided they can meet the necessary criteria regarding vaccination and identification.

To enter the UK without quarantine from a listed or EU country, dogs and cats must have a PETS passport or certificate containing information on the animal:

- Permanently identified with an electronic microchip
- Vaccinated against rabies using an inactivated vaccine
- Have an official health certificate containing details of:
  - owner or keeper
  - identification and description of animal
  - vaccination record and booster information
  - blood tests and results
  - treatment for ticks and tapeworms

If an animal arrives in the UK and does not meet the PETS requirements (see Chapter 6) the authority responsible for carrying out the checks will decide, in consultation with the owner and a veterinary surgeon, whether to re-export the animal; to put it into quarantine (possibly for up to six months) until it can comply with the PETS rules; or, as a last resort, to put the animal down.

Quarantine for six months on arrival in the UK should be pre-arranged before travelling begins from an unlisted country. Official transporters collect animals on arrival from ports and airports. On arrival at the quarantine premises the animal is taken to its allocated unit. It cannot be moved to any other unit during its stay unless there is an emergency or the move is approved by the attending veterinary surgeon.

All animals are given appropriate accommodation according to size and species. There are recommended minimum internal measurements for individual units, which also state sleeping area and adjoining exercise area size.

Guidelines are in place for the general standards of hygiene, materials used on surfaces in quarantine kennels (e.g. non-slip floors). Also stated are feeding and management routines, the need for visual stimuli and fresh air access, the condition and minimum temperature of the sleeping area.

The animal's owner is allowed reasonable access for visiting during the six-month quarantine period. If any signs of ill health arise during the quarantine, the attending veterinary surgeon is consulted and the owner of the animal is informed immediately.

Appendix
Anatomy and Physiology Terminology

The majority of terms referring to the body systems and medical conditions are derived from Greek or Latin. Most of these terms are a combination of two or more word parts. When they combine to become a word, they usually indicate some or all of the following:

- Body tissues involved
- What has gone wrong
- Quantity (a lot or very little)
- Levels of infection or inflammation
- Colour or substance
- Fluid involved

You may find it helpful to practise defining the components of the words separately, then combine them to find out the meaning of the complete word. In many ways it is no different from learning a new language and by memorising the common beginnings and endings, the rest can be worked out. It is always helpful to have a veterinary dictionary for the less frequently used terms and words.

Medical terminology

Certain syllables are commonly used as the beginning or ending of medical terms, in many cases being added to a word stem which refers to a particular organ or part of the body.

- *Prefix* – beginning of a word stem
- *Suffix* – ending of a word stem

Prefixes in anatomy/physiology

A or **An** – lack of, e.g. anaemia (lack of blood cells)
Dys – difficult or defective, e.g. dysphagia (difficulty swallowing)
Endo – within, e.g. endoscope (equipment used to look at working organs)
Ex – out, e.g. excision (to remove)

Haema or **Haemo** – refers to blood, e.g. haemorrhage (loss of blood)
Hyper – excess of, e.g. hyperthermia (high body temperature)
Hypo – lack of, e.g. hypothermia (low body temperature)
Poly – many or much, e.g. polydipsia (drinking a lot)
Pyo – pus, e.g. pyometra (pus-filled uterus)
Sub – beneath or under, e.g. sublingual (under the tongue)

Suffixes in anatomy/physiology

itis – inflammation, e.g. arthritis (inflammation of a joint)
logy – science or study of, e.g. dermatology (study of the skin)
penia – deficiency, e.g. leucopenia (deficiency of white blood cells)
phagia – eating, e.g. coprophagia (eating faeces)
rrhoea – increased discharge, e.g. diarrhoea (increased discharge of faeces)

Word use

The following common words may help to illustrate the prefix/suffix idea:

- *Nephritis* – **neph** refers to the specialised cell of the kidney, known as the nephron; **itis** refers to inflammation of a tissue. The meaning of this word is kidney cell inflammation and pain.
- *Arthritis* – **arth** refers to a joint; **itis** means inflammation. The meaning of this word is joint inflammation and pain.
- *Hepatitis* – **hepat** refers to the specialised cell of the liver know as the hepatocyte; **itis** means inflammation. This word means inflammation and pain of the liver cells.
- *Haematoma* – **haem** refers to blood; **toma** refers to a lump or swelling. The meaning of this word is blood-filled lump or swelling.

These words are descriptions, not diagnoses, and simply refer to a tissue type or organ and what is happening to it.

Anatomical directions

Anatomical directions are used to describe areas of the animal body. They are part of the language of medicine used between colleagues for communication. Many of these words originated from Greek or Latin.

The first four words are another way of saying above, below, front and back and are in common use when case recording in the medical world:

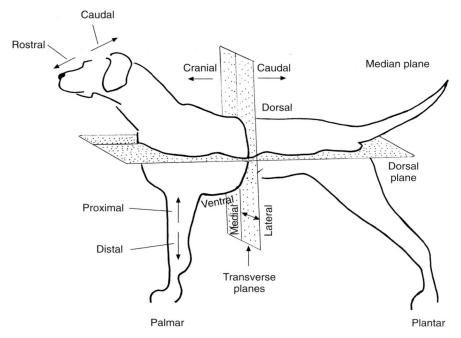

Fig. A.1 Anatomical diections. Adapted from McBride, D.F. (1996) *Learning Veterinary Terminology*. Mosby, St Louis.

- *Dorsal* – towards the top or back surface of the body
- *Ventral* – towards the underside, lower surface or nearer the ground
- *Cranial or anterior* – situated at the front of the body or towards the head end
- *Caudal or posterior* – situated towards the back end of the body or towards the tail

Words to indicate side, middle or near the nose are:

- *Lateral* – to the side (left or right) or away from the middle of the body
- *Medial* – the midline of a body structure or the body
- *Rostral* – on the head but towards the nose

Words indicating near or far from a named body structure (especially limbs) are:

- *Proximal* – near to the body trunk or closer to a named structure
- *Distal* – away from the body trunk or further from a named structure

Words which describe where on a limb, surface, especially lower limb, surfaces are:

- *Palmar or volar* – indicating the caudal or back surface of the fore-limb, below the carpus or wrist area
- *Plantar* – indicating the caudal or back surface of the hind limb, below the tarsus or hock area

Words indicating inside or outside are:

- *Internal* – inside the body
- *External* – outside or surface

Selected Reading

SECTION 1

Animal Science

Beckett, B.S. (1993) *Biology*. Oxford University Press, Oxford.
Blood, D.C. & Studdert, V.P. (1998) *Comprehensive Veterinary Dictionary*. Baillière Tindall, London.
Clegg, C. (1990) *Biology*. Heinemann, Oxford.
Jones, G. (1991) *Biology*. Cambridge University Press, Cambridge.
Lane, D. & Cooper, B. (1999) *Veterinary Nursing*. Pergamon Press, Oxford.
Michell, A.R. & Watkins, P.E. (1989) *Introduction to Veterinary Anatomy and Physiology*. BSAVA, Cheltenham.
Roberts, M.B.V. (1995) *Biology: A Functional Approach*. Nelson, London.

Genetics

Grossman, A. (1992) *The Standard Book of Dog Breeding*. Doral, Wilsonville, USA.
Nicholas, F.W. (1991) *Veterinary Genetics*. Oxford Science, Oxford.
Taylor, D. (1986) *You and Your Dog*. Dorling Kindersley, London.
Taylor, D. (1986) *You and Your Cat*. Dorling Kindersley, London.

SECTION 2

Ackerman, D.L. (n.d.) *Cat Health*. TFH, USA.
Alderton, D. (1986) *Rabbits and Guinea Pigs – Petkeeper Guide.* Salamander, London.
Alderton, D. (1989) *The Dog Care Manual*. Stanley Paul.
Anderson, R.S. & Edney, A.T.B. (1990) *Practical Animal Handling*. Pergamon Press, Oxford.
Barrie, A. (1987) *Step by Step – Guinea Pigs*. TFH, USA.
Bell, J.C., Palmer, S.R. & Payne, J.M. (1988) *The Zoonoses*. Edward Arnold, London.
Burger, I. (1993) *The Waltham Book of Companion Animal Nutrition*. Pergamon Press, Oxford.
Colville, J. (1991) *Diagnostic Parasitology for Veterinary Technicians*. American Veterinary Publications, California.
Dallas, S. & Simpson, G. (1999) *Manual of Veterinary Care*. BSAVA.
Evans, J.M. & White, K. (1994) *Book of the Bitch*. Henston, Guildford.
Evans, J.M. & White, K. (1994) *The Catlopaedia.* Henston, Guildford.
Evans, J.M. & White, K. (1994) *The Doglopaedia.* Henston, Guildford.

Fletcher, N. (2000) *Essential Guide to Fish Care*. Internet Publishing.

Fox, S. (1988) *Rats*. TFH, USA.

Harkness, J.E. & Wagner, J.E. (1985) *The Biology and Medicine of Rabbits and Rodents*. Lea & Febiger, Philadelphia.

Henwood, C. (1990) *Step by Step – Hamsters*. TFH, USA.

Lane, D. & Cooper, B. (1999) *Veterinary Nursing*. Pergamon Press, Oxford.

McCurnin, D.M. (1994) *Clinical Text for Veterinary Technicians*. W.B. Saunders, Philadelphia.

Morris, D. (1986) *Animal Watching*. Jonathan Cape, London.

Richardson, V.C.G. (1992) *Diseases of Domestic Guinea Pigs*. Blackwell Science, Oxford.

Thies, D. (1989) *Cat Care*. TFH, USA.

SECTION 3

Bell, C.T.P. (1993) *First Aid and Health Care for Dogs*. Lutterworth Press, Cambridge.

Edney, A.T.B. & Hughes, I.B. (1986) *Pet Care*. Blackwell Science, Oxford.

Fogle, B. (1995) *First Aid for Dogs*. Pelham, London.

Kirk, R.W. & Bistner, S.I. (1985) *Handbook of Veterinary Procedures and Emergency Treatment*. W.B. Saunders, Philadelphia.

Lane, D. & Cooper, B. (1999) *Veterinary Nursing*. Pergamon Press, Oxford.

McBride, D.F. (1996) *Learning Veterinary Terminology*. Mosby, St Louis.

Taylor, D. (1986) *You and Your Cat*. Dorling Kindersley, London.

Taylor, D. (1986) *You and Your Dog*. Dorling Kindersley, London.

Index